The Paramedic
Revision Guide

David W. Thom

Specialist Practitioner - Critical Care, Dorset and Somerset Air Ambulance, Henstridge, Somerset, UK

WILEY Blackwell

Registered Office(s)
John Wiley & Sons, Inc., 111 River Street, Hoboken, NJ 07030, USA
John Wiley & Sons Ltd, The Atrium, Southern Gate, Chichester, West Sussex, PO19 8SQ, UK

Editorial Office
9600 Garsington Road, Oxford, OX4 2DQ, UK

For details of our global editorial offices, customer services, and more information about Wiley products visit us at www.wiley.com.

Wiley also publishes its books in a variety of electronic formats and by print-on-demand. Some content that appears in standard print versions of this book may not be available in other formats.

Library of Congress Cataloging-in-Publication Data

Names: Thom, David W., author.
Title: The paramedic revision guide / David W. Thom.
Description: First edition. | Hoboken, NJ : Wiley-Blackwell, 2021. |
   Includes bibliographical references and index.
Identifiers: LCCN 2021008650 (print) | LCCN 2021008651 (ebook) | ISBN
   9781119758068 (paperback) | ISBN 9781119758075 (adobe pdf) | ISBN
   9781119758082 (epub)
Subjects: MESH: Emergency Medicine | Anatomy | Physiological Phenomena |
   Emergencies | Pharmacology | Evidence-Based Practice
Classification: LCC RC86.8 (print) | LCC RC86.8 (ebook) | NLM WB 105 |
   DDC 616.02/5–dc23
LC record available at https://lccn.loc.gov/2021008650
LC ebook record available at https://lccn.loc.gov/2021008651

Cover Design: Wiley
Cover Image: © Stone's Throw Media/Shutterstock

Set in 9.5/12pt Myriad by SPi Global, Pondicherry, India
Printed and bound by CPI Group (UK) Ltd, Croydon, CR0 4YY

C9781119758068_200521

Disclaimer

The information included within this book is written with the best intention and knowledge at the time; however, some of the content may be out-of-date at the time of reading. Local guidelines, procedures and national variation may affect the application of this text in practice. Local guidance should be adhered to in line with your employer's policy. The author accepts no responsibility for the actions or omissions of individuals. Practise only within the scope of practice as designated by your employer and professional registration. This book is designed as a study aid and further reading may be required. Every effort has been made to identify and reference the information within this book. Any omissions or inaccuracies are not intentional and will be rectified upon notifying the publisher.

Contents

Preface

This book is designed to take some of the mystery out of the education for paramedics, a handy go-to text for students, professionals and educators alike. The aim of this book is to provide the basis to understand the key areas of paramedic sciences and practice.

The reason for developing this book was to provide a different option away from the heavy clinical textbooks with the goal of providing succinct and easily digestible information. This should help not only with the stress of exams during the training period of being a paramedic but also throughout your career as a professional as a handy reference tool.

Paramedicine as a profession has developed in leaps and bounds since the early days of its inception. Not only are paramedics and pre-hospital clinicians performing at a level that would seem far-fetched only a decade or so ago but now the profession has extended beyond the realms of solely working on a 999-response vehicle. Extended scope, specialist and advanced practice are all now very much within the grasp of paramedics. However, understanding the basics of the profession is the key to developing a core knowledge base on which to build.

Although titled for paramedics, most of the underpinning themes and knowledge cross professional boundaries with other allied health professionals and the nursing profession. I hope that this text is of use to any and all that read it.

Since the introduction of undergraduate higher education for paramedics, there has been more emphasis on the academic abilities of a paramedic, I hope that this book will help guide your revision and study throughout your training and career.

1

Paramedic anatomy and physiology – 1

Contents

This section will take you through the basics of anatomy, physiology and some pathophysiology required for your learning. Physiology is often overlooked but it underpins every aspect of clinical care within medicine. By understanding the physiology you can interpret how the patient is presenting even if you don't know what is wrong with them, from this you will be able to form management plans to alter the physiology back to normal.

Firstly what you will need to learn is how to classify areas of the body and general terms for describing movement and positioning within healthcare. It may seem daunting at first but with repetition and application in practice the terms will stick. There are regular question breaks throughout to check your learning.

The Paramedic Revision Guide, First Edition. David W. Thom.
© 2021 John Wiley & Sons Ltd. Published 2021 by John Wiley & Sons Ltd.

Anatomical and medical terms

2

Anatomy – The science of the body structures and the relationship between them studied by dissection.
Physiology – The science of how the body functions and the actions of each organ.
The anatomical position – Facing forwards with palms forwards

Regions of the body

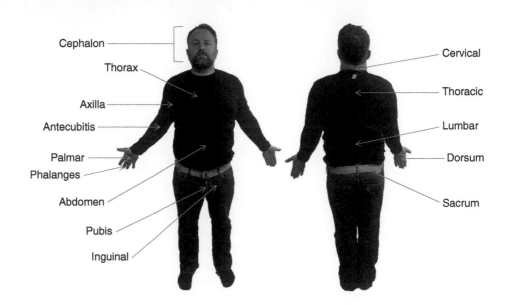

Figure 1.1 A labeled representation presented in the anatomical position.

Directional terminology

Superior – Above or higher to the point described e.g. the head is superior to the shoulders
Inferior – Below or lower to the point described e.g. the bowel is inferior to the diaphragm
Anterior (Ventral) – Towards the front of (using the anatomical position) e.g. the sternum is anterior to the heart.
Posterior (Dorsal) – Towards the back of e.g. the oesophagus is posterior to the trachea
Medial – Closer to the midline e.g. the heart is medial to the lungs
Lateral – Further from the midline e.g. the lungs are lateral to the heart
Ipsilateral – On the same side as e.g. the gallbladder and the appendix are ipsilateral
Contralateral – On the opposite side to e.g. the spleen is contralateral to the ascending colon
Proximal – Closer to the point of origin e.g. the knee is proximal to the ankle
Distal – Further from the point of origin e.g. the wrist is distal to the elbow
Superficial – Closer to the surface e.g. the epidermis is superficial to the subcutaneous
Deep – Further below the surface e.g. the subcutaneous is deep to the epidermis

Anatomical planes

Midsagital – Divides the body or organ vertically into *equal* left and right portions
Parasagital – Divides the body or organ vertically into *unequal* left and right portions
Frontal (Cronal) – Divides the body or organ vertically into anterior and posterior portions
Transverse – Divides the body or organ horizontally into superior and inferior portions
Oblique – Passes through the body or an organ at an angle

Postural terms

Supine – Lying on their back
Prone – Lying on their front
Right lateral recumbent - Lying on their right side
Left lateral recumbent - Lying on their left side
Fowlers – Sitting up with legs bent or straight
Tredelenburg – Lying supine with their legs raised

> These terms, although it may not seem it now, are essential to your practice as they allow for greatly improved paperwork, handovers and conversations with colleagues.

Planes of movement

A**b**duction – Movement away from the midline e.g. raising arms out (to abduct)
A**dd**uction – Movement towards the midline e.g. lowering arms (to add together)
Flexion – Bending at a joint e.g. raising forearm (flexing biceps)
Extension – Straightening a joint e.g. lowering forearm (extending a hand to shake)
Medial rotation – Turning inwards e.g. toe in
Lateral rotation – Turning outwards e.g. toe out
Supination – Rotation of the forearm so that the palm faces forwards (palm UP)
Pronation – Rotation of the forearm to that the palm faces backwards (palm DOWN)

Abdominal regions

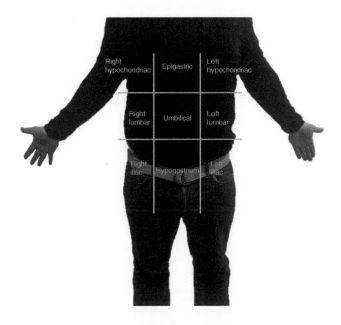

Figure 1.2   Labeled nine regions of the abdomen.

Questions

1. Without looking, define the following terms. (These you can check yourself)
   a. Anterior
   b. Proximal
   c. Inferior
   d. Medial
   e. Superficial
2. Fill in the blanks
   a. The kidneys are _____ to the stomach
   b. The shoulders are _____ to the head
   c. The trachea is _____ to the oesophagus
   d. Brain is found in the _____ region
   e. The fingers are _____ to the wrist
3. A patient found lying on their back is said to be in what position?
4. The plane that divides the body or an organ vertically into equal left and right portions is what?
5. What movement is involved when the hand touches the shoulder?

Further questions – don't worry if you can't answer these now you may choose to research these now, but if not be sure to revisit them later.

6. The appendix is found in which region? (Try to use the nine segments)
7. Trendelenburg position is primarily utilised in patients with what?
8. Shortening and lateral rotation of a leg is a sign of (but not definitively) what?

> The last few pages have been very wordy so here are some questions just to help test if it has gone in. See what you can do without looking.

> Answers can be found at the back of the book

References and Further Reading

Gregory, P. and Ward, A. (2010). *Sanders' Paramedic Textbook*. Edinburgh: Mosby Elsevier.

Marcovitch, H. (2017). *Black's Medical Dictionary*, 43e. London: Bloomsbury.

Tortora, G.J. and Derrickson, B.H. (2017). *Tortora's Principles of Anatomy and Physiology*, 15e. Chichester: Wiley.

Waugh, A. and Grant, A. (2018). *Ross and Wilson Anatomy and Physiology*. Edinburgh: Elsevier.

Cellular biology

Nice to know or need to know? This may seem a bit in depth for a Paramedic however having a good understanding at this level allows for a greater understanding on a larger scale. The benefits will also show when discussing drugs later on! Let's start with the basics.

Cells are complicated but the basics can be broken down at this level. We will build on this throughout the book so it's worth getting an understanding now. So what makes up a cell?

Parts of a cell

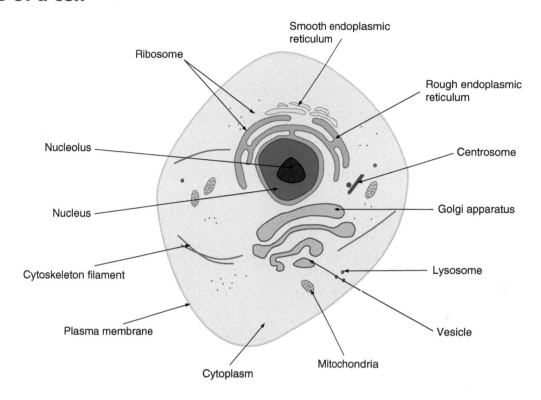

Figure 1.3   Labeled diagram of a cell.

The cell wall

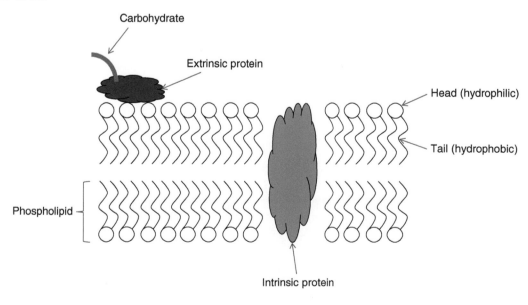

Figure 1.4   Simplified depiction of the phospholipid bilayer of a cell wall.

Functions of the main organelles

- Nucleus – Storage and synthesis of DNA
- Mitochondria – Production of energy in the form of ATP (Adenosine triphosphate) by respiration
- Rough Endoplasmic Reticulum – Protein synthesis
- Smooth Endoplasmic Reticulum – Lipid synthesis
- Centrioles – Microtubules associated with nuclear division
- Golgi apparatus – Storage, modification and packaging of proteins and other chemicals

Biological terms

Diffusion – The movement of substances from an area of *high* concentration to *low* concentration.

Facilitated diffusion – The movement of substances from an area of *high* concentration to *low* concentration using a carrier protein or protein channel.

Osmosis – The movement of *water* from an area of *high* concentration to *low* concentration through a semi-permeable membrane. (Only refers to water).

Active transport – The movement of substances **against** the concentration gradient using energy (i.e. area of **low** concentration *to* an area of **high** concentration).

Tissue

Tissues can be classified into four main groups.

1. Epithelial e.g. skin
2. Connective tissue e.g. ligaments
3. Muscle e.g. bicep
4. Nervous e.g. neurons

However epithelial tissue is further divided into:

1. Squamous – Thin and flat
2. Cuboidal – Cube shaped
3. Columnar – Column structure
4. Simple – Single layer
5. Stratified – Multi-layered cells
6. Ciliated – Possess cilia (the so-called 'hairy' cells)

So why is this important? Well understanding what the organelles do allows you to work out what may be affected if they stop functioning correctly. Classification of cells is especially important as it allows you to gain a better knowledge of how larger areas work, for example the Mucociliary escalator in the trachea.

Quick Questions

Cover up the previous information and answer the following statements with true or false.

1. The smooth endoplasmic reticulum synthesises protein.
2. The blood is an example of connective tissue.
3. Diffusion is the movement of water from an area of *high* concentration to *low* concentration.
4. Human cells contain a cell wall.
5. The tail of the cells in the phospholipids bilayer is hydrophilic.

References and Further Reading

Alberts, B., Johnson, A., Lewis, J. et al. (2015). *Molecular Biology of the Cell*, 6e. Abingdon: Garland Science.
Gregory, P. and Ward, A. (2010). *Sanders' Paramedic Textbook*. Edinburgh: Mosby Elsevier.
Tortora, G.J. and Derrickson, B.H. (2017). *Tortora's Principles of Anatomy and Physiology*, 15e. Chichester: Wiley.
Waugh, A. and Grant, A. (2018). *Ross and Wilson Anatomy and Physiology*. Edinburgh: Elsevier.

The nervous system

The nervous system is often a complex part of the anatomy to discuss at it has many different aspects and its functions are widespread. This section will try to break it down into easy to digest sections.

Feedback systems

The nervous system uses feedback systems in order to maintain homeostasis. Homeostasis is defined as equilibrium in the body's internal environment. This is done by constant interaction from the body's many regulatory processes.
   Feedback systems have three sections

1. Sensory
2. Control centre
3. Effectors

Negative feedback systems *reverse* a change in a controlled condition e.g. the body's internal temperature. When the temperature is too high the body dilates peripheral circulation and increases sweating amongst other methods.

Positive feedback systems *strengthen* or *reinforce* a change in a controlled condition for a better outcome e.g. labour. When there is pressure applied to the cervix by the foetus during labour the body releases *oxytosin* which induces cervical dilation. This increases until the pressure is relieved by the baby being born.
   The major functions of the nervous system are to:

1. Send and receive *sensory* functions
2. Send and receive *motor* functions
3. Integrate information
   a. Storage of information
   b. Analysis of information
   c. Decision making

The nervous system can be divided into its major sections as follows.

- Brain
- Brain stem
- Cranial nerves
- Spinal cord
- Central nervous system
- Peripheral nervous system

The brain has four lobes:

- Frontal
- Parietal
- Temporal
- Occiptal

The brain also encompasses the cerebellum and brainstem

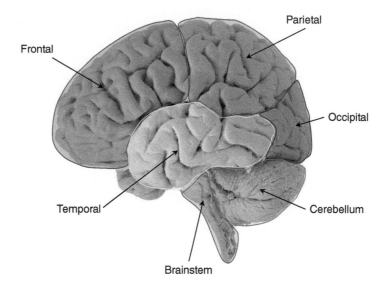

Figure 1.5 Labeled diagram depicting the regions of the brain.

Neuronal anatomy

The central nervous system refers to the brain and spinal cord. It integrates information from the peripheral nervous system. The peripheral system consists of everything outside of the brain and spinal cord.

Nervous tissue consists of two main types

1. Neuroglia
2. Neurones

Neuroglia assists the nervous system in *maintaining homeostasis*

Table 1.1 Denoting the difference in neuroglia between the central and peripheral nervous system.

Neuroglia in the central nervous system	Neuroglia in the peripheral nervous system
Astrocytes • Metabolise neurotransmitters • Assist impulse transmission • Form the blood–brain barrier	Satellite cells • Support neurones in ganglia
Oligodendrocytes • Form myelination	Schwann cells • Form myelination
Microglia • Phagocytic cells	
Ependymal cells • Ciliated for assisting movement of Cerebrospinal fluid	

Neurons carry the impulses to and from the brain and have three main types

1. Unipolar
2. Bipolar
3. Multipolar

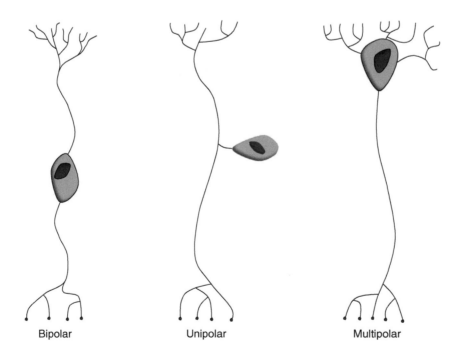

Bipolar   Unipolar   Multipolar

Figure 1.6 Simplified depiction of neurons.

Definitions

Stimulus – Change in the environment (internal or external) that is strong enough to create an action potential.

Action potential – The ability to respond to stimuli with an electrical impulse.

Threshold – A point that when reached or surpassed by a stimulus releases an action potential.

Afferent – sensory, carries an action potential towards the central nervous system.

Efferent – motor, carries an action potential away from the central nervous system.

Remember S.A.M.E. Sensory is Afferent, Motor is Efferent

Myelination

1. Electrical insulation of the neuron
2. Increases speed of impulse conduction

Conduction of impulses

Continuous

- *Non*-myelinated neurones.
- Domino effect. As sodium flows in during depolarisation the neighbouring gates open.
- Refractory period prevents the conduction from travelling backwards.

Saltatory

- Occurs in myelinated neurones.
- Impulse 'jumps' between Nodes of Ranvier.
- Allows for faster conduction.

Resting cell membrane potential and conduction in the average neuron

1. Rests at −70 mV.
2. Depolarises to +30 mV.
3. Returns to resting.

Why do you need to know this? At this level, it may seem a bit much but at level two you are able to administer drugs that affect this process so having a good understanding now makes it easier.

Action potential response to stimulus

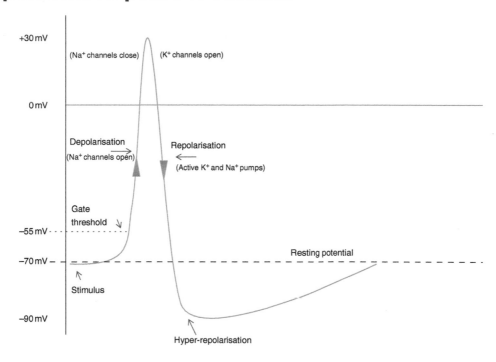

Figure 1.7   Diagram demonstrating the electrical response (action potential) to a stimulus.

Conduction

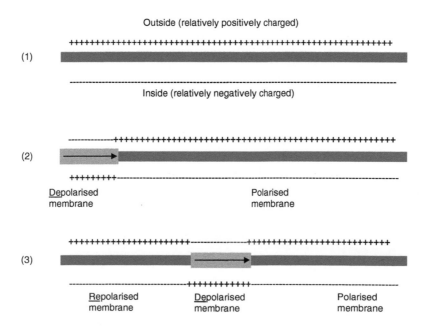

Figure 1.8   Visual representation of propagation of an impulse along a cell membrane.

Speed of impulse propagation

The speed of propagation is dependent on the strength of the impulse.
   Factors that increase the speed of propagation are:

- Larger diameter fibres
- Myelination
- Warmer temperatures

Synapses

Electrical

- Found in the heart
- Current spreads through *gap junctions*
- Allows for synchronised conduction to achieve co-ordinated contraction
- Two way unlike a chemical synapse, this helps explain how an impulse can travel 'backwards' in the heart.

Chemical

- Occur where two neurones meet
- The gap between them is bridged by neurotransmitters
- A neurotransmitter is released when an action potential reaches the axon bulb forcing the chemicals to be released into the synapse by exocytosis.
- Neurotransmitter is received by a receptor on the postsynaptic bulb
- Here, an action potential can be stimulated or blocked
- One-way impulse conduction

Neurotransmitters

- Work to open or close specific ion channels
- Some work slowly by secondary messenger systems
- Result in excitation or inhibition of postsynaptic neuron
- Many are hormones secreted by endocrine organs

This bit is probably in the nice to know section at this stage but definitely worth a read

Examples of neurotransmitters

1. Acetylcholine – used in the Parasympathetic nervous system (this will be covered later) can be affected by organophosphate overdoses
2. Epinephrine – Adrenaline used for fight or flight responses
3. Dopamine – creates feeling of elation. This can be affected by illicit drugs such as cocaine
4. Gamma Aminobutyric Acid (GABA) – affected by diazepam
5. Serotonin – patients may be on Selective Serotonin Reuptake Inhibitors (SSRI's)
6. Enkephalins and Endorphins – Released by exercise, chocolate etc.

Questions

1. Fill in the blanks
   a. Myelinated neurones use _____ conduction
   b. Feedback systems require the following functions; sensory, _____ and _____.
   c. An _____ neuron carries impulses away from the Central Nervous System

We're not done on the nervous system yet, but here are some questions to test what you know so far

2. Answer the next statements with True or False
   a. Temperature control is an example of positive feedback
   b. The axon contains the cell nucleus
   c. An action potential is the ability to respond to a stimuli with an electrical impulse
   d. Chemical synapses are two way
3. What forms the myelin sheath in the Central Nervous System?
4. What factor can be utilised by a paramedic to increase the effectiveness of analgesia?

The cerebrum

Is the most superior part of the brain and consists of two main areas

1. Cortex, which is the outer layer consisting of grey matter (Non-mylenated)
2. Medulla, which is the inner layer consisting of white matter (Mylenated)

The cerebrum is divided into left and right hemispheres by the **Falx Cerebri** which is an extension of the **Dura Mater.**
   The three principal functions are

1. Mental activity
2. Sensory perception
3. Control of voluntary muscle

The Cerebrum contains basal ganglia that are groups of neurones that assist in the control of large automatic movements. These are affected in patients suffering from Parkinson's.
   The limbic system is located in the Cerebrum and Diencephalon and controls the emotional aspects of behaviour related to survival. It also plays a role in memory.
   There are ventricles in the brain containing cerebral spinal fluid.

1. Lateral – One in each cerebral hemisphere
2. Third – Between and inferior to the left and right hemisphere
3. Fourth – Between the brain stem and cerebellum

The cerebellum

Controls the skeletal muscle contractions required for

- Balance
- Posture
- Skilled movements
- Muscle tone

Compares the intended movement with the actual movement

Diencephalon

Thalamus

- 80% of the diencephalon
- Relays all sensory information to cerebral cortex
- Crude appreciation of senses; e.g. pain, heat so that it can be directed to appropriate areas of the brain

Hypothalamus

- Controls and integrates with the Autonomic Nervous system
- Associated with rage and aggression
- Regulates
  - Body temperature
  - Fluid intake via thirst centre
  - Food intake via feeding and satiety centres
  - Waking and sleeping patterns associated with the reticular activating system
- Connects nervous system and endocrine systems

The brain stem

Midbrain

- Approximately 2.5 cm in length (In the average adult)
- Connects the Pons to the Diencephalon
- Carries Motor impulses to and from the spinal cord to cerebrum and cerebellum
- Directs impulses
- Origin of Cranial Nerves III and IV

Pons Varolii

- Approximately 2.5 cm in length (In the average adult)
- Connects spinal cord to the brain
- Links various areas of the brain
- Pneumotaxic area
  - Shortens inspiratory phase to increase respiration rate
- Apneustic area
  - Lengthens expiratory phase to decrease respiration rate
- Origin on Cranial Nerves V–VII

> These are important to know as it allows you to work out how a patient may present if one of these areas is affected e.g. a brain stem CVA.

Medulla Oblongata

- Approximately 2.5 cm in length (In the average adult)
- Contains the Pyramids of Decussation which cross the neuron paths
- Contains the following
  - Cardiac centre - control of the cardiac muscle
  - Respiratory centre - control aspects of breathing
  - Vasomotor centre – control of vascular tone e.g. vasoconstriction
- Possesses reflex centres for; coughing, sneezing, hiccupping, swallowing, vomiting, etc.
- Origin of Cranial Nerves VIII–XII
- Cranial nerve X is the Vagal nerve

Spinal cord

The Spinal cord has three protective coverings called meninges, these also extend over the brain. These are called the Dura mater, Arachnoid mater and the Pia mater. The spinal cord terminates at the superior border of L2 where it becomes the Cauda Equina.

Dura mater

- Outermost covering made of dense connective tissue
- Stops expansion of brain and spinal cord

Arachnoid mater

- Middle layer made from a web of collagen fibres
- Avascular (without blood, oxygen and nutrients are provided by the Cerebrospinal fluid)
- CSF circulates in Sub-Arachnoid space

Pia mater

- Innermost layer made from thin transparent connective tissue
- Contains blood vessels

In the spinal cord, white mater surrounds the grey mater centre, the opposite of the brain.

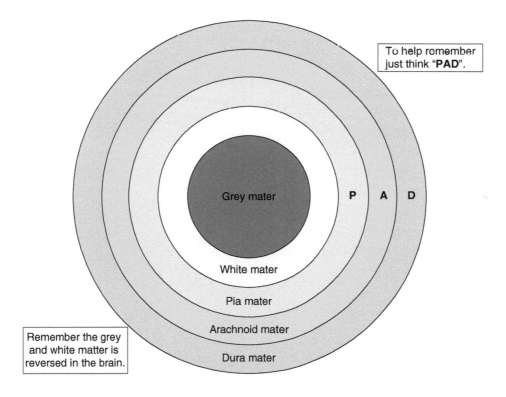

Figure 1.9 Visual representation of the layers of the spinal cord.

Spinal cord functions

1. Anterior portion controls motor nerves
2. Posterior portion controls sensory nerves

3. Links brain to the peripheries
   a. Relays messages entering and leaving at the same level
   b. Relays messages entering and leaving at different levels
   c. Relays messages to and from the brain
4. Acts as centre for reflex action

Reflex arc

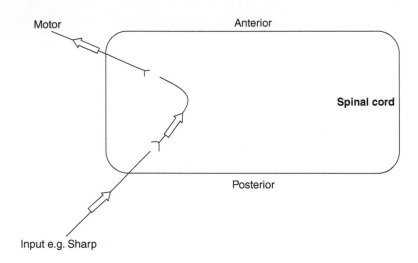

Figure 1.10   Simplified diagram of a spinal reflex arc.

Cortical reflex

Follows the spinal reflex to

- Reinforce, modify or inhibit reaction
- Apply the appropriate response e.g. swearing

Autonomic reflex

- No conscious control e.g. rises in blood pressure resulting in vasodilatation etc.
- Can occur independently or in conjunction with other systems to maintain homeostasis

Important nerves

- The Phrenic nerve leaves the spinal cord at C3–5
- The Cardiac nerves leave the spinal cord at T1–4
- The Intercostal nerves leave the spinal cord at T2–12

> Remember the phrase '**Three, four and five keeps you alive'** and you will never forget the phrenic nerve!

Cerebrospinal fluid (CSF)

The CSF is formed in the ventricles of the brain by filtration of the blood plasma, a process done by the Choriod Plexuses. An average adult has approximately 80–150 mL of circulating fluid which is re-absorbed at a rate of 20 mL/hour by the arachnoid villi and venous dural sinuses.

Its main functions are

- Mechanical protection
  - Cushions tissues from being damaged by cranial and vertebral bones
- Chemical protection
  - Optimal environment for hormonal activity
  - Changes in the CSF can affect neurotransmitters
- Circulation
  - Medium for the exchange of nutrients and waste substances

Peripheral nervous system

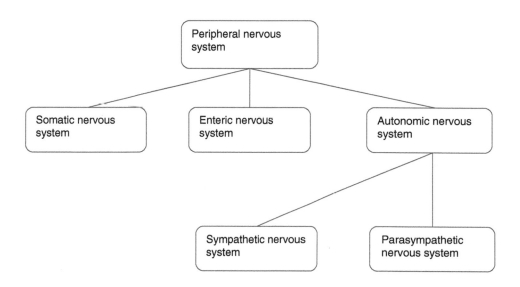

Figure 1.11 Diagram denoting the facets of the peripheral nervous system.

Somatic nervous system

- From the muscle to the CNS
- Sensory neurones and proprioceptors
- Proprioceptors detect movement to allow brain to estimate where the limb is in relation to the body in addition to rigorous, e.g. exercise, movement stimulating the respiratory centre to keep up with an increased oxygen demand.

Enteric nervous system

- 'Brain of the gut'
- Controlled by Enteric Plexuses
- Work, to an extent, separate from the Central and Autonomic Nervous systems
- Communicate with the CNS by parasympathetic neurones
- Monitor changes e.g. Chemical levels in the Gastrointestinal tract

18

Autonomic nervous system

- Network of sensory neurons all over the body
- No conscious control
- Maintains homeostasis
- Controls; blood pressure, blood flow, body temperature, digestion, respiration, etc.
- Sub-divided into the Sympathetic and Parasympathetic nervous systems

Sympathetic nervous system

- Known as the '**accelerator**'
- Expends energy
- Mainly uses Epinephrine and Norepinephrine as neurotransmitters
- Leaves from the spinal cord

Parasympathetic nervous system

- Known as the '**brake**'
- Conserves energy
- Mainly uses Acetylcholine as a neurotransmitter
- Leaves from the brainstem and sacrum

Effects of the autonomic nervous system

Ciliary muscle

- Ring of smooth muscle holding the lens in the eye
- Receives only Parasympathetic innervations
- Acetylcholine (ACh) causes constriction to allow for near vision

Iris

- Receives both Sympathetic and Parasympathetic innervations
- Parasympathetic causes pupil to constrict (Miosis)
- Sympathetic causes pupil to dilate (Mydriasis)

Heart

- Receives both Sympathetic and Parasympathetic innervations
- Parasympathetic innervates the Sinoatrial node to induce bradycardia
- Parasympathetic nervous system does *not* innervate the myocardium
- Sympathetic innervates all regions of the heart
  - Increases rate at Atrioventricular node
  - Increases conduction through the purkinjee fibres
  - Increases force of ventricular contraction
- A young healthy heart is dominated by Vagal tone

Respiratory

- Receives both Sympathetic and Parasympathetic innervations
- Parasympathetic evokes constriction of smooth muscle leading to bronchoconstriction
- Sympathetic evokes dilation of smooth muscle leading to bronchodilation

Gastrointestinal

- Receives both Sympathetic and Parasympathetic innervations
- Normally dominated by parasympathetic tone
- Parasympathetic nervous system causes increased gut motility
- Sympathetic causes a reduction in cut motility

Urinary Bladder

- The Detruser muscle is controlled by the parasympathetic
- The Trigone muscle is controlled by the sympathetic

It is important to understand the role of the autonomic nervous system, as it will help you understand more about the physiology of a patient's condition. It will also help you when we move on to talk about drugs you might give later on.

Think of the Autonomic Nervous system in terms of the fight or flight response. For example, you are walking home alone at night and you decide to take the shortcut down a dark alley. In the alley, you are confronted by a mad axe man who states he is going to kill you (doesn't seem like such a good idea anymore does it?). The Sympathetic or 'Accelerator' kicks in which results in:

- Pupil dilation as you want to be able to see where you are going so you don't trip over
- Increased heart rate as you want the blood circulating faster so you can run away
- Arties dilate improving blood supply to skeletal muscle so that you can run faster
- Bronchi dilate as you need to breathe easily to continue running
- GI tract decreases in motility as you don't want to defecate yourself (that would just be embarrassing)
- Bladder, well that works roughly in the same sense as the GI tract.

Table 1.2 Effects of nervous system innervation on the sympathetic and parasympathetic nervous system.

Effect of nervous innervations on	Sympathetic	Parasympathetic
Eye	Dilation of pupils and relaxation of lens for enhanced vision	Constriction of pupils and contraction of lens for near vision
Heart	Increased heart rate, contractility and conduction velocity	Decreased heart rate, contractility and conduction velocity
Arterial system	Constrict most blood vessels, dilates vessels to; heart, lungs and skeletal muscle	Supply very few vessels for vasodilatation
Bronchi	Relaxes bronchial smooth muscle and inhibits the secretion of mucus	Contracts bronchial smooth muscle and stimulates the secretion of mucus
Stomach	Decreases the motility and keeps the sphincters closed	Increases the motility and opens the sphincters
Bladder	Relaxes bladder wall and contracts the sphincter	Contracts the bladder wall and relaxes the sphincter

Questions

1. Fill in the blanks
    a. The cortex is the _____ layer of the cerebrum
    b. The most superior part of the brainstem is the _____
    c. Directly inferior to that is the _____
    d. The most inferior part of the brainstem is the _____
    e. The _____ nerve leaves at level C3-5
    f. The _____ nervous system is known as the 'brain of the gut'
2. Answer the statements with True or False
    a. The cerebrum contains the reflex centres for vomiting and coughing
    b. The hypothalamus is the largest part of the diencephalon
    c. The vagus nerve originates in the medulla oblongata
    d. Sympathetic stimulation with case a decrease in the motility of the stomach and the opening of the sphincters
3. Where are the Pyramids of Decussation found?
4. Name the three meninges of the brain and spinal cord.
5. How much circulating Cerebrospinal fluid does the average adult have?

References and Further Reading

Alberts, B., Johnson, A., Lewis, J. et al. (2015). *Molecular Biology of the Cell*, 6e. Abingdon: Garland Science.

Crossman, A.R. and Neary, D. (2019). *Neuroanatomy*, 6e. London: Elsevier.

Gregory, P. and Ward, A. (2010). *Sanders' Paramedic Textbook*. Edinburgh: Mosby Elsevier.

Lou, L. (2015). *Principles of Neurobiology*. London: Taylor and Francis Group.

Tortora, G.J. and Derrickson, B.H. (2017). *Tortora's Principles of Anatomy and Physiology*, 15e. Chichester: Wiley.

Waugh, A. and Grant, A. (2018). *Ross and Wilson Anatomy and Physiology*. Edinburgh: Elsevier.

The respiratory system

Respiratory complaints are a common presentation to the ambulance service, therefore, understanding the basic anatomy and physiology will help with your understanding of the disease process. This section will not look at illnesses in detail as this will be covered later.

Components

1. Nose
2. Pharynx
3. Larynx
4. Trachea
5. Bronchi
6. Bronchioles
7. Terminal Bronchioles
8. Alveolar Ducts
9. Alveoli
10. Lungs

Nose

- External
  - Bone and Hyaline cartilage covered by muscle and skin
  - Two openings (Nares) separated by the septum
  - Lined with mucous and hairs
- Internal
  - Large cavity in skull
  - Inferior to cranium, superior to mouth
  - Merges the external nares to the pharynx
  - Lateral walls make from; Ethmoid, Maxillae, Lacrimal, Palatine and inferior Conchae bones
  - Roof formed if Palatine bones
  - Contains three 'shelves' formed by projection of nasal chonchae
  - Highly vascular
- Functions
  - Warm air
  - Moisten air
  - Filter air
  - Receive olfactory stimulus
  - Resonating chamber for speech sounds

These two are probably a nice to know but still useful

Pharynx

- Funnel-shaped tube approximately 13 cm long in the average adult
- Extends from the internal nares to the cricoids cartilage
- Skeletal muscle with mucous membrane
- Supplied by cranial nerves IX, X, and XI
- Separated into three parts the Nasopharynx, Oropharynx and the Laryngopharynx

Nasopharynx

- Extend from nares to level of soft palate
- Five openings
  - Two external nares
  - Two Eustachian tubes
  - One opening to Oropharynx
- Pharangeal tonsil on posterior wall (adenoid)
- Functions
  - Receive air from internal nares
  - Equalise pressure in the ears, nose and throat
  - Filters dust-laden particles

Oropharynx

- Extends from soft palate to level of hyoid bone
- Lined with stratified squamous epithelium
- Contains Palatine and Lingual Tonsils

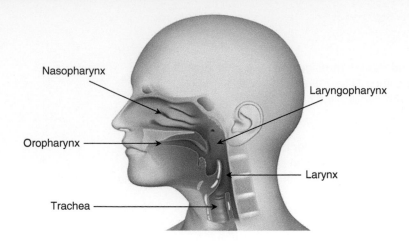

Figure 1.12   Labeled diagram of the upper airway.

Laryngopharynx

- Most inferior portion of pharynx
- Opens into
  - Oesophagus (posterior)
  - Larynx (anterior)
- Lined with stratified squamous epithelium

Larynx

- Contains nine pieces of cartilage
- Single cartilage
  - Thyroid
  - Epiglotis
  - Cricoids
- Paired cartilage
  - Arytenoids
  - Corniculate
  - Cuneiform
  - Glottis

> At this level understanding, the Larynx contains nine pieces of cartilage should be sufficient. However, it will help in a later section where these will be studied in greater detail. It will also be covered when discussing Endotracheal Intubation.

Trachea

> Don't get too concerned with the measurements, as everyone is individual.

- *Approximately* 12 cm in length in the average adult
- *Approximately* 2.5 cm in diameter in the average adult
- 16–20 'C' shaped cartilages incomplete posterior to allow food passage down the oesophagus
- Lined with pseudo stratified ciliated columnar epithelium
- Mucociliary Escalator 'wafts' Mucous towards pharynx for expulsion

Bronchi

- Bifurcate from the Trachea at the Carina at the level of T5
- The right main bronchus is shorter, wider and more vertical than the left
- Composed of incomplete rings of hyaline cartilage and pseudo stratifies ciliated columnar epithelium

- On entry to the lungs at the Hilum they split into the secondary bronchi
- These then divide into tertiary bronchi
- These then divide into the bronchioles
- Cartilage is gradually replaced by smooth muscle in the bronchioles

Bronchioles

- Are to respiration what arterioles are to circulation
- Varying the diameter controls the air movement
- Divide into terminal bronchioles

Alveoli

- Approximately 150 million in the average adult
- Allow gas exchange between the blood and air
- Use natural surfactants to stop them from collapsing and sticking
- Increase surface area in the lungs

Lungs

- Right lung has three lobes
- Left lung has two lobes due to the cardiac notch
- Surrounded by the pleura which has two layers
  - Visceral pleura attaches to the lung to allow smooth expansion
  - Parietal pleura anchors the lungs to the chest wall
  - Space in-between in known as the pleural cavity
  - Can become infected and cause pleuritis or pleurisy
  - Fluid entering the pleural cavity is known as *pleural effusion*

Knowing the definition of these terms and the volumes is important in aiding your understanding of the patient's conditions. Also, it will help guide your treatment if you understand the physiological processes going on.

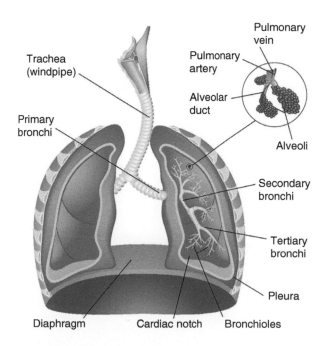

Figure 1.13   Labeled diagram of the respiratory tract.

Respiratory processes

Pulmonary Ventilation

- Mechanical flow of air in and out of the lungs

External Respiration

- Exchange of gasses from the alveoli to the blood and back again

Internal Respiration

- Exchange of gasses between blood and tissues

Pulmonary volumes

Tidal volume

- Normal air inhaled and exhaled during normal breathing
- Approximately 500 mL in the average adult

Inspiratory reserve volume

- Largest additional volume that can be forcibly inhaled above tidal
- Approximately 3100 mL in the average adult

Expiratory reserve volume

- Largest additional volume that can be forcibly exhaled above tidal
- Approximately 1200 mL in the average adult

Residual volume

- Amount of air that cannot be forcibly exhaled from the lungs
- Approximately 1200 mL in the average adult

Vital capacity

- Largest volume of air that can be inhaled and exhaled from the lungs in one go
- Approximately 4800 mL in the average adult

Dead air space

- Amount of air left in conducting airways
- Approximately 150 mL in the average adult

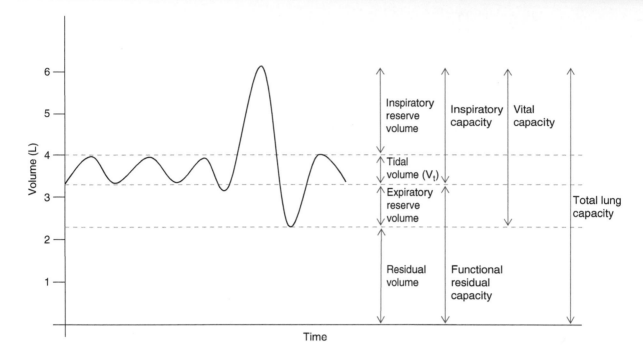

Figure 1.14   Example spirograph annotated.

Total lung capacity

- Amount of air that can be held in the lungs
- Approximately 6000 mL in the average adult

Breathing

Breathing is the movement of air in and out of the lungs. This is done by creating a pressure gradient by the movement of the diaphragm and the ribs. On inhalation, the pressure in the lungs is lower than atmospheric air so air moves into the lungs. On exhalation, the pressure in the lungs is greater than atmospheric air so the air is drawn out again.

The relevance of this is that naturally we breathe by negative pressure; however, when you are ventilating your patient you will use positive pressure. What effect might this have? What about if they have a pneumothorax?

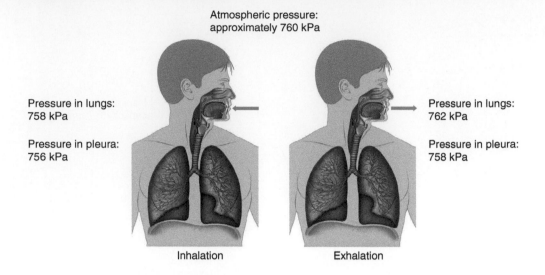

Figure 1.15   Pressure changes during inhalation and exhalation.

Exchange

This takes place due to pressure gradients within the body. These are created by differing Partial pressures (p) of gasses.

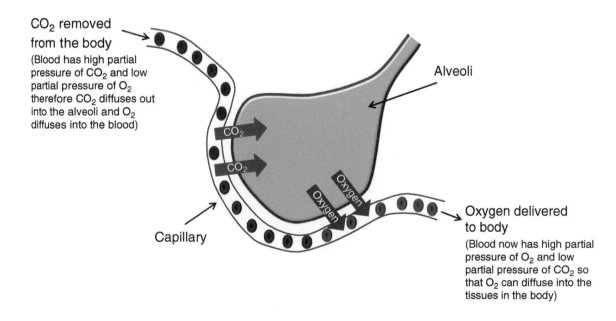

Figure 1.16   Gas exchange within the alveoli.

Questions

1. Fill in the blanks
   a. The Pharynx is supplied by cranial nerves _____, _____ and _____.
   b. The trachea bifurcates at the _____.
   c. The average expiratory reserve volume is _____.
   d. Normal breathing requires _____ pressure.
2. Answer the following statements with True of False
   a. The nose has external and internal sections
   b. The trachea contains 16–20 'C' shaped cartilages incomplete anterior to allow food passage down the oesophagus
   c. The right lung has three lobes
3. Why is the right main bronchus more prone to blockage?
4. Define external respiration.

Regulation

- Breathing is regulated by nervous control and chemical regulation.
- Nervous control is regulated by the respiratory centres in the brainstem.
- Chemical regulation is controlled by the chemoreceptors.
  - When there is a rise in pCO_2 in the blood it stimulates the brainstem to induce breathing.

In patients with advanced Chronic Obstructive Pulmonary Disease (COPD) the body's chemoreceptors can become accustomed to a higher level of CO_2 in the blood and, therefore, less responsive. As a result, in a small cohort of patients, breathing will be stimulated by a reduction the in concentration of oxygen in the blood. This can be referred to as the *Hypoxic Drive*.

Hypoxia

Note: This does not apply to Paraquat poisoning
Defined as: low oxygen at tissue level.
Hypoxic Hypoxia

- Low levels of oxygen in the arteries

Anaemic Hypoxia

- Reduced functioning haemoglobin (Hb) in the blood. This could be due to haemorrhage, anaemia, etc.

Stagnant Hypoxia

- Inability for blood to carry oxygen to the tissues in order to support their needs. This could be due to clots of cardiac problems.

Histoxic Hypoxia

- Inability of cells to adequately us the delivered oxygen e.g. cyanide poisoning.

Gas laws

Boyle's Law

> These gas laws are important not only because they will come up on your exam but they allow you to understand explain the pathophysiology of conditions to a far greater detail as well as the treatments.

- The pressure within a close container varies *inversely* with the size of the container.
  - The bigger the container the lower the pressure if filled with the same amount of gas.

Dalton's Law

- At a constant temperature and volume, the total pressure exerted by a mixture of gasses is equal to the sum of the partial pressures.

Henry's Law

- The quantity of gas that will dissolve in a liquid is *proportional* to the partial pressure of the gas and the solubility coefficient.
  - Greater pp + greater solubility coefficient = Greater solubility

Charles's Law

- The same gas will occupy different volumes at different temperatures
  - Increase the temperature = increased volume

> Unfortunately, as yet, I have not found an easy way to remember these; it will just take some time to learn. When they are used in practical demonstrations later they should make more sense.

Quick Questions

1. How is breathing regulated?
2. What are the four types of hypoxia?
3. What is Cole's law?
4. What is it called when all or part of the lung collapses?
5. Describe the three processes of the respiratory system

References and Further Reading

Bersten, A.D. and Handy, J.M. (2018). *Oh's Intensive Care Manual*. Edinburgh: Elsevier.

Bourke, S.J. and Burns, G.P. (2015). *Respiratory Medicine: Lecture Notes*, 9e. Chichester: Wiley Blackwell.

Gregory, P. and Ward, A. (2010). *Sanders' Paramedic Textbook*. Edinburgh: Mosby Elsevier.

Tortora, G.J. and Derrickson, B.H. (2017). *Tortora's Principles of Anatomy and Physiology*, 15e. Chichester: Wiley.

Waugh, A. and Grant, A. (2018). *Ross and Wilson Anatomy and Physiology*. Edinburgh: Elsevier.
West, J.B. and Luks, A.M. (2015). *West's Respiratory Physiology*, 10e. Alphen aan den Rijn: Wolters Kluwer.

The cardiovascular system

The cardiovascular system can be thought of in three main groups; the blood, the blood vessels and the heart. Each group has further divisions.

Table 1.3   Components of the cardiovascular system.

Blood	Blood vessels	Heart
Red Blood Cells (RBC)	Arteries	Coronary circulation
White Blood Cells (WBC)	Arterioles	Pulmonary circulation
Platelets	Capillaries	Systemic circulation
Plasma	Venules	
	Veins	

Table 1.4   Role of the blood.

Transportation	Protection	Regulation
Dissolved substances	Clotting	pH
Nutrients	Against infection	Body temperature
Hormones		Water content of cells
Waste products		

Blood

Functions:
- Blood is a connective tissue consisting of a liquid matrix
- Equates for approximately 8% of body weight in the average adult
- Blood temperature is approximately 38 °C
- Blood pH is between 7.36 and 7.44
- Formed in *red* bone marrow at a rate of 2 mL/second on average

Erythrocytes

- Bi-concave shape for an increased surface area
- Mature cells have no nucleus
- Contain Haemoglobin which is a quaternary structure protein surrounding and Iron molecule
- Carry oxygen in the blood

Leukocytes

- Play a vital role in the body's immune response
- Can be granular or agranular
- Formed in spleen, liver, lymph nodes and red bone marrow

Thrombocytes (platelets)

- Smaller than other formed elements
- Produced in the bone marrow
- Vital for clotting in the blood

Blood groups

Each erythrocyte has antigens on the cell membrane; it is these antigens that determine the blood group. The blood also contains antibodies for other antigens just like infections.

When a person is given the wrong type of blood it can lead to **agglutination** by the antibodies. For example, if a patient with blood group A were given blood from a group B donor this would lead to agglutination. Because type O blood had no antigens, it is known as the universal donor and as patients with AB blood have no antibodies against either antigen they are known as the universal recipient.

A patient's blood is considered positive or negative depending if there is a Rhesus antigen present. If it is present the blood is considered positive.

Table 1.5 Correlation between blood group and blood antibodies.

Blood group	Antibody's in blood
A	Anti-B
B	Anti-A
AB	None
O	Anti-A and Anti B

Clotting cascade

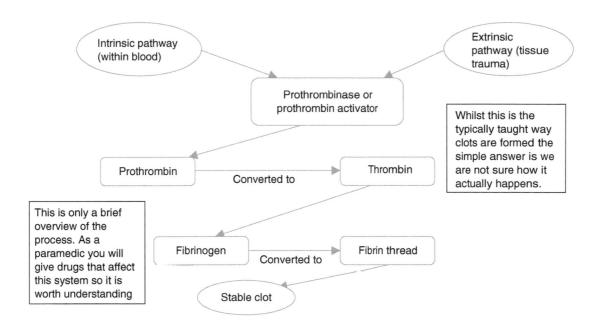

Figure 1.17　Simplified clotting cascade.

Blood vessels

Arteries

- Carry oxygenated blood away from the heart (with the exception of pulmonary circulation)
- Strong outer layer (**Tunica Adventitia** or externa)
- Thick muscular middle layer (**Tunica Media**)
- Smooth inner lining (**Tunica Intima** or interna)
- Great internal pressure
- Utilises elastic recoil to assist in the movement of blood
- Contains roughly 13% if blood volume
- Anastomoses are branches between arteries or arterioles to provide an alternate route for blood
- End arteries contain no anastomoses so if blocked will shut off blood supply to an area e.g. the finger

Arterioles

- Microscopic in size
- Regulate blood supply by the use of sphincters

Capillaries

- Allow the transfer of products in and out of the fluid
- More prolific in areas of high metabolic activity e.g. the liver

Venules

- Connect blood supply from the capillaries to the veins

Veins

- Carry deoxygenated blood towards the heart (with the exception of pulmonary circulation)
- Thick outer layer
- Thinner middle layer
- Smooth inner layer
- Larger lumen than arteries
- Contain valves to prevent backflow of blood
- Contain approximately 65% of circulation blood

Pulmonary circulation

Pulmonary circulation works at a much lower pressure than systemic circulation to allow for gas exchange to take place. The pulmonary circulation holds about 10% of the body's blood volume.

Pulmonary arteries

- Carry deoxygenated blood from the right ventricle to the lungs
- Enter the lungs at the hilum
- Low-pressure system

Pulmonary veins

- Carry oxygenated blood from the lungs into the left atria
- Two from each lung

Systemic circulation

- Works at a much higher pressure have the left ventricle is more muscular
- Oxygenated leaves the left ventricle via the Aorta
- Systemic circulation holds about 85% of the body's blood volume

Coronary circulation

- Coronary circulation is filled during diastole of the heart. This is because during systole the Aortic valve covers the opening to protect the vessels from the high pressures
- Left coronary artery splits into the anterior interventricular artery and the circumflex
- Right coronary artery splits into the posterior interventricular artery and the marginal

Questions

1. Fill in the blanks
   a. Patients with type A blood have anti-_____ antibodies
   b. The three main functions of the blood are: _____, _____ and _____.
   c. Oxygenated blood leaves the left ventricle via the _____.
2. Answer the following statements with True or False
   a. Blood is slightly acidic
   b. Fingers contain arteries with no anastomoses
   c. All veins carry deoxygenated blood
   d. The left coronary artery splits into the anterior interventricular branch and the circumflex
3. What are the five main types of blood vessel?
4. When does the Coronary circulation fill?
5. Why?

The heart

Location

- Sits at the approximate level of T4/T5
- Sits *media sternum* (between the lungs)
- Rests on sternum and diaphragm
- Cardiac spinal nerves originate between T1–T4

Although these locations are approximate you can imagine if there is damage to any of these structures it may result in cardiac issues.

Three distinct layers

- *Peri*cardium
- *Myo*cardium
- *Endo*cardium

Pericardium

Has three distinct layers

Pericardium

- One outer layer made of dense fibrous tissue attaches the heart to the diaphragm
- Two inner layers
    - Outer *parietal* is fused to the outer pericardium
    - Inner *visceral* adheres to the myocardium
- Between the two inner layers is a thin film of serous fluid to allow for smooth contraction of the heart by reducing friction

Myocardium

- Involuntary muscle
- Each cell/fibre is in contact with its immediate neighbour
- Electrical impulses pass between cells by the use of gap junctions
- Can act independent to the autonomic nervous system
- Myocardial cells contain large levels of mitochondria to produce the energy needed

Endocardium

- Innermost layer of the heart
- Smooth non-stick layer to reduce friction on the blood
- Continuous endothelium with the blood vessels

Parts of the heart

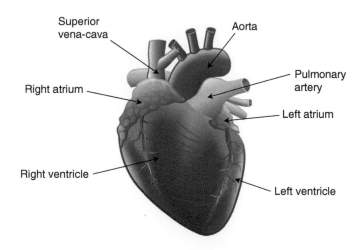

Figure 1.18   Labeled heart.

Flow through the heart

Table 1.6 Flow through the heart.

Right atrium	*Left atrium*
1. Deoxygenated blood from vena cava and coronary sinus 2. Sinoatrial node 3. Atrioventricular node 4. Baroreceptors 5. Tricuspid valve into the RV	1. Oxygenated blood from four pulmonary veins 2. Baroreceptors 3. Bicuspid valve into the LV
Right ventricle	*Left ventricle*
1. Separated from atrium by thick connective insulating tissue 2. Separated from left ventricle by thick muscular septum 3. Pumps blood into pulmonary circulation 4. Pulmonary Semi-lunar valve into the pulmonary artery	1. Separated from atrium by thick connective insulating tissue 2. Pumps blood into systemic and coronary circulation 3. Myocardium is 50–100% thicker than right ventricle 4. Aortic Semi-lunar valve into the Aorta

Cardiac terminology

Systole

- Contraction of the cardiac muscle

Diastole

- Relaxation of the cardiac muscle

End systolic volume

- Volume of blood left in the ventricles after contraction

End diastolic volume

- Volume of blood in the ventricles at full diastole

Isovolumetric contraction

- The point in the cardiac cycle where the ventricles are contracting but all the valves are closed

Cardiac output

- Amount of blood ejected from the ventricles into circulation

Stroke volume

- Amount of blood ejected from the left ventricle every beat
- In men, it averages at 70 mL and in women the average is 80 mL

Preload

- Amount of blood in the ventricle before contraction

Afterload

- Amount of pressure the heart must overcome to eject the blood into circulation

Fluid dynamics in capillaries

There are many forces that determine the movement of fluid from the blood vessels. The basic principles are that if the pressure within the vessel then fluid will pass through into the interstitial fluid and onto the cells. When the pressure falls the flow is reversed to allow the removal of waste products.

Physiology, and more so pathophysiology, can affect this. By reducing the pressure on the arterial side then less is able to pass **into** the interstitial fluid thus reducing the perfusion to the cells. If the patient has high osmotic pressures then more fluid is drawn from the interstitial fluid affecting the distribution and perfusion to the cells. There are also oncotic pressures to be considered but this will become more important later when discussing pathologies such as sepsis or ketoacidosis.

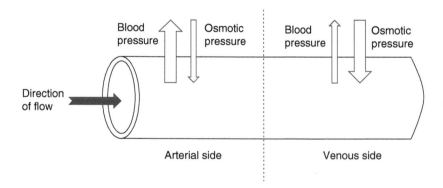

Figure 1.19   Simplified diagram of fluid dynamics.

Conduction system

The electrical impulses in the heart are created by action potentials and, in a normal heart, travel through specific routes.

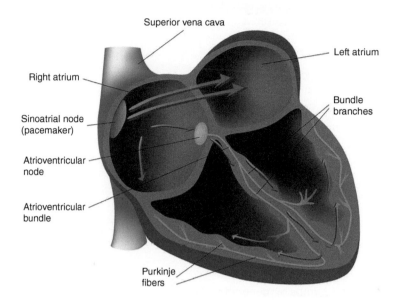

Figure 1.20   Labeled conduction system of the heart.

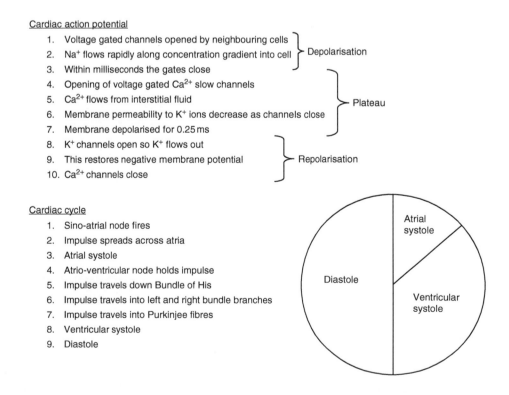

Cardiac action potential

1. Voltage gated channels opened by neighbouring cells ⎫
2. Na⁺ flows rapidly along concentration gradient into cell ⎬ Depolarisation
3. Within milliseconds the gates close ⎭
4. Opening of voltage gated Ca^{2+} slow channels
5. Ca^{2+} flows from interstitial fluid
6. Membrane permeability to K⁺ ions decrease as channels close ⎬ Plateau
7. Membrane depolarised for 0.25 ms
8. K⁺ channels open so K⁺ flows out
9. This restores negative membrane potential ⎬ Repolarisation
10. Ca^{2+} channels close

Cardiac cycle

1. Sino-atrial node fires
2. Impulse spreads across atria
3. Atrial systole
4. Atrio-ventricular node holds impulse
5. Impulse travels down Bundle of His
6. Impulse travels into left and right bundle branches
7. Impulse travels into Purkinjee fibres
8. Ventricular systole
9. Diastole

Figure 1.21   Representation of the proportional time takes during a cardiac cycle.

Cardiac laws

Frank-Starling law states that if you increase the preload on the heart you will increase the stretch and the volume. This is associated with the Bainbridge reflex, which uses baroreceptors in both atria and the aortic and carotid bodies to detect the stretch. When there is too great a stretch they stimulate the cardiac centre to alter the body e.g. decrease heart rate or vasodilatation.

Marey's law states that the heart rate will increase if a low blood pressure is detected. The body uses this law as a compensatory mechanism.

There has been a lot covered so far which may be quite heavy but will start to make sense as it is applied to practice.

Questions

1. Fill in the blanks
    a. Contraction of the cardiac muscle is known as _____
    b. Atrial contraction is indicated by the _____ wave
2. Answer the following statements with true or false
    a. The heart has three distinct layers
    b. The right ventricle pumps oxygenated blood
    c. The visceral pericardium attaches to the myocardium
3. Where is the heart situated?
4. Where do the cardiac nerves leave the spinal cord?
5. Define the electrical pathway through the heart
6. What is isovolumeteric contraction?

Electrocardiogram (ECG)

The ECG is used to show the electrical activity in the heart; however, it may not correlate to the mechanical action undertaken by the heart. It can be used as a diagnosis tool for many common conditions. At this level, we will focus on the basics of ECG.

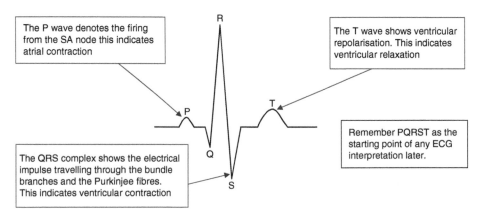

Figure 1.22   Example ECG complex.

Getting the basics right on a 'simple' rhythm strip will help with interpretation later. At this level, you should keep things simple. Here are the few simple things to look for.

1. Is there a trace?
   a. This might seem simple but making sure the leads are attached is the first step
2. Is it regular or irregular?
   a. On a separate sheet of paper mark the point of 3 complexes and slide along, the following complexes should line up
   b. If it is irregular is it regularly irregular?
      i. Beat, beat, pause, beat, beat, pause, beat, beat (regularly irregular)
      ii. Beat, pause, pause, beat, beat, beat, beat, pause (irregularly irregular)
3. What is the heart rate?
   a. Count the number of LARGE squares between two 'R' points then divide by 300 to give you a rough rate. (This only works with regular rhythms)
4. Is there a 'P' wave before every 'QRS'
5. Is there a 'QRS' after every 'P' wave
6. Can you feel a pulse with every QRS

At this stage, this is all you need to think about with ECG's. Try not to over complicate things too early on as it will be easier with experience and seeing more.

Basic ECG traces

We will cover ECG's in more detail in section two but here are the basics.

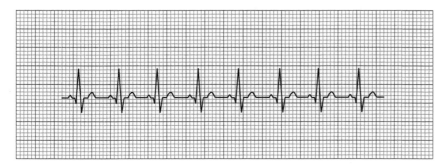

Normal Sinus Rhythm. QRS follows every P wave

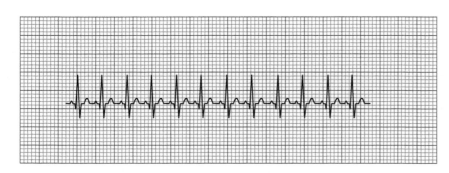

Sinus Tachycardia (rapid rate)

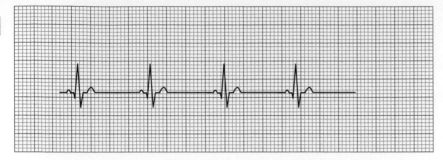

Sinus Bradycardia (slow rate)

Atrial Fibrillation. No P waves with a chaotic baseline

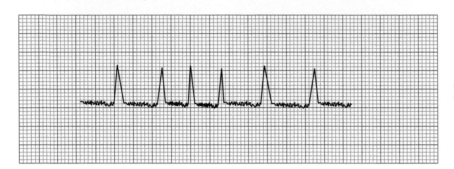

Heart block

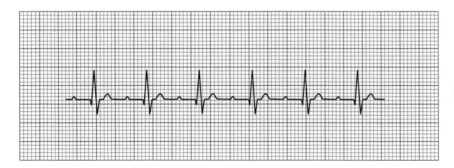

1st degree AV block
Lengthening of PR interval

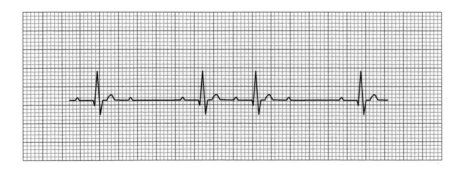

2nd degree (type 1) AV block.
P waves with intermittent dropped QRS complex

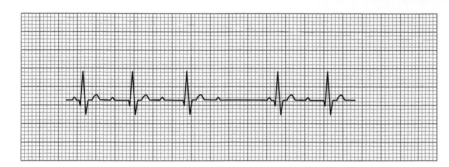

2nd degree (type 2 - Wenckebach) AV block. Lengthening PR interval before dropped QRS

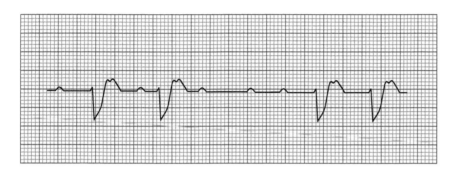

3rd degree (complete) AV block. Total disassociation between P waves and QRS.

When the Atrial complex (P wave) can't get through) the myocytes in the ventricles generate and electrical impulse and contraction. This is why the QRS appears different in 3rd-degree block.

Cardiac emergencies

These will need to be learned for the Advanced Life Support OSCE's and for practice.

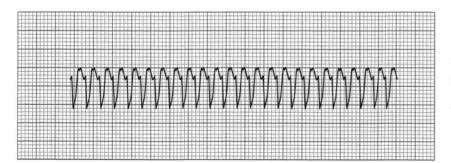

Ventricular tachycardia (VT). If the patient does <u>NOT</u> have a pulse (unless trained) then it **CAN be shocked i.e. cardiac arrest**

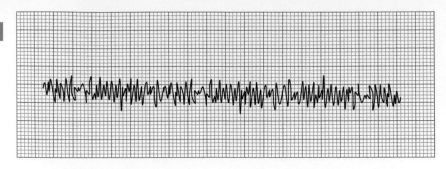

Ventricular Fibrillation (VF).
Chaotic with no discernable
complexes **SHOCKABLE
RHYTHM**

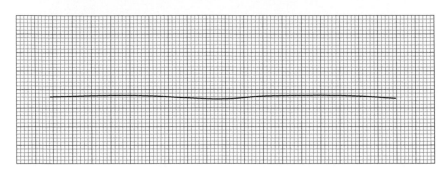

Asystole
This is **NON**-shockable

References and Further Reading

Gregory, P. and Ward, A. (2010). *Sanders' Paramedic Textbook*. Edinburgh: Mosby Elsevier.

Hampton, J. and Hampton, J. (2019). *The ECG Made Easy*, 9e. Edinburgh: Elsevier.

Herring, N. and Paterson, D.J. (2018). *Levick's Introduction to Cardiovascular Physiology*, 6e. London: CRC Press.

Life In The Fast Lane (2021). https://litfl.com/ecg-library/basics/.

Peate, I. and Nair, M. (2016). *Fundamentals of Anatomy and Physiology: For Nursing and Healthcare Students*, 2e. Chichester: Wiley Blackwell.

Tortora, G.J. and Derrickson, B.H. (2017). *Tortora's Principles of Anatomy and Physiology*, 15e. Chichester: Wiley.

Waugh, A. and Grant, A. (2018). *Ross and Wilson Anatomy and Physiology*. Edinburgh: Elsevier.

The gastrointestinal system

Food is broken down in the body by mechanical and chemical processes this starts in the mouth and ends at the rectum.

Food travels in the following order:

Mouth → Oesophagus → Cardiac sphincter → Stomach → Pyloric sphincter → Duodenum → Small intestine → Ascending colon → Transverse colon → Descending colon → Sigmoid colon → Rectum

Let's look at some of the parts individually:

Stomach

- Initial digestion of food
- Uses **acid** and mechanical churning
- Acids neutralise some bacteria

Duodenum

- Food exits the stomach into the duodenum
- Food mixes with bile from gallbladder
- Digestive juices from pancreas mix here

Small intestine

- Nutrient and mineral absorption
- Bacteria break down food
- **Alkali** conditions
- Food moved through using peristalsis (wave-like motion)
- Microscopic finger-like projections called villi increase surface area

Large intestine

- Water and other substances absorbed
- Vitamins such as vitamin K created by bacteria and absorbed
- Waste products formed into stool for defecation
- May become inflamed and cause colitis

Liver

- Separated into lobes
- Has certain ability to heal/regenerate itself unlike any other body part
- Bile production
- Excretion of bilirubin, hormones
- Filtration and excretion into the gallbladder of drugs
- Metabolism of fats, proteins, and carbohydrates
- Enzyme activation for metabolism
- Storage of glycogen, vitamins, and minerals
- Synthesis of proteins such as albumin and clotting factors
- Removal of toxins from blood
- Heat generation
- Can become damaged through trauma, medications, alcohol, drugs or other poisons (natural or man-made)

This will become important when we go on to discuss drugs later on.

Gallbladder

- Collection and concentration of bile
- Bile is created by the liver and biliary tract using waste products and specialised cells
- Bile is then secreted into the intestinal tract
- If the biliary tree, gall bladder or outflow tract becomes blocked this can cause biliary colic, cholecystitis (inflammation of the gall bladder) and even liver failure as the liver is unable to excrete waste products.
- Drugs such as the contraceptive pill are excreted into the gallbladder and then into the intestines where it is re-absorbed. This is called enterohepatic reuptake. (this one is nice to know and not need to know at this level)
- Can become inflamed causing cholecystitis

Pancreas

- Produces enzymes for digestion
- Produces hormones such as insulin
- Retroperitoneal (behind the peritoneum)
- Can become inflamed causing pancreatitis

Spleen

- Recycles red blood cells
- Storage of blood products such as white blood cells
- Immune system response
- Can become damaged in trauma causing bleeding

Appendix

- Uncertain function
- May have some use in the immune response
- Can become inflamed and cause Appendicitis

Peritoneum

- Thick covering that surrounds most of the organs in the abdomen except the kidneys and most of the pancreas
- Can become inflamed and cause peritonitis normally as a response to other infections/inflammations
- Secures the placement of organs as well as provide protection

References and Further Reading

Gregory, P. and Ward, A. (2010). *Sanders' Paramedic Textbook*. Edinburgh: Mosby Elsevier.

Peate, I. and Nair, M. (2016). *Fundamentals of Anatomy and Physiology: For Nursing and Healthcare Students*, 2e. Chichester: Wiley Blackwell.

Tortora, G.J. and Derrickson, B.H. (2017). *Tortora's Principles of Anatomy and Physiology*, 15e. Chichester: Wiley.

Waugh, A. and Grant, A. (2018). *Ross and Wilson Anatomy and Physiology*. Edinburgh: Elsevier.

The endocrine and exocrine system

The endocrine system consists of glands that are spread throughout the body and have no physical connection to each other. A gland is a cell or group of cells that are specially adapted to excrete products.

In the endocrine system uses capillary networks to facilitate the wider diffusion of these chemicals closely surround them. These chemicals can also be known as hormones, which are a chemical messenger.

These hormones can provide a local or widespread effect by only affecting the cells with the appropriate receptors.

The greater the number or receptors on a cell the greater effect the hormone will have

The endocrine can work **in addition to** the nervous system to *enhance* or *alter* a change in the body.

- Autonomic nervous system provides a rapid change
- Endocrine systems provide a slower but more precise change with a longer lasting effect

Hormone types

Steroid Hormone

- Amino acid derivative
- Peptide hormone
- Carried in the bloodstream weakly bound to plasma proteins, when bound they can exert no effect
- Insoluble in water but soluble in lipids
- Generally ac within the nucleus

Non-Steroid Hormone

- First messenger system
- After binding to a receptor it activates the G-protein
- The G-protein activates Adenylatecyclose or other proteins

> This much depth shouldn't be expected of you at this level but understanding they cause a chain reaction is.

Prostaglandins

- *Paracrine* substances (**act locally**)
- Exert a multitude of effects on the body
  - Intensifying pain
  - Inflammation
  - Fever
  - Smooth muscle tone
  - Glandular secretions
  - Blood flow
  - Reproductive systems
  - Platelet function
  - Nerve impulse transmission
  - Immune response

> Understanding the roles that prostaglandins have in body is essential, as you will be administering drugs that exert their effect at his level.

Hormone secretion

Hormone secretion is controlled in three basic ways within the body.

- Hypothalamus controls the pituitary glands and the release of tropic hormones
- Nervous system can provide direct stimulus to the glands
- Direct glandular response to changes in the internal environment

Glands

- 1 pituitary gland anterior to the hypothalamus
- 1 pineal gland posterior to the hypothalamus
- 1 Hypothalamus
- 1 thyroid gland
- 2 ovaries or testis
- 4 parathyroid glands
- Multiple pancreatic islets
- 2 adrenal glands
- 1 thymus gland

The pancreas

The pancreas contains both endocrine and exocrine functions.
  Endocrine

- Secretion of Glucagon (alpha cells)
  - Promotes conversion of glycogen to glucose in the liver
  - Promotes glyconeogenisis which is the production of glucose from other substances in the body
  - Stimulated by blood glucose levels
  - Example of a negative feedback system
- Secretion of Insulin (beta cells)
  - Promotes conversion of glucose to glycogen in the liver and skeletal muscle
  - Promotes carbohydrate metabolism
  - Stimulated by blood glucose levels
  - Stimulates protein synthesis
- Secretion of Somatostatin (delta cells)
  - Inhibits production of Glucagon and Insulin
  - Slows rate of food absorption and enzyme secretion in the gut

Exocrine

- Produces pancreatic juices to neutralise stomach acid in duodenum
- Secreted into bile duct

Adrenal glands

Medulla (centre)

- Produces Epinephrine
- Produces Norepinephrine

Cortex (outer layer)

- Produces Glucocorticoids e.g. Cortisol
  - Regulate metabolism and respond to stress
  - Cortisol is the most abundant hormone
  - Promotes lipolysis
  - Anti-inflammatory properties
  - Involved in the immune system and depression
- Produces Mineral corticoids e.g. aldosterone
  - Involved in the maintenance of homeostasis
  - Aldosterone used in the maintenance of blood pressure
- Produces sex steroids e.g. testosterone
  - Involved in puberty and muscle tone

Regulation of blood pressure

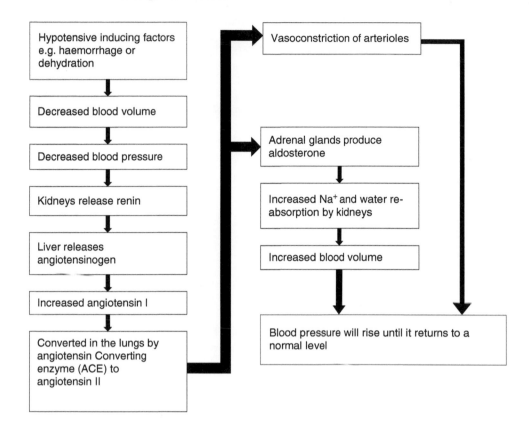

Figure 1.23   Renin-angiotensin cycle.

Understanding how the body regulates blood pressure is essential as patients will regularly be on medication that will affect parts of this system. For example patients may be on Ramipril, which is an ACE inhibitor. How might this affect blood pressure? Why might they be on it?

Questions

1. Fill in the blanks
    a. The stomach is highly _____
    b. Steroid hormones are _____ derivative
    c. The _____ of the adrenal glands produces epinephrine
    d. Ramipril works to _____ blood pressure
2. Answer the following statements with true or false
    a. The gallbladder is situated in the right hypochondriac region
    b. The endocrine portion of the pancreas produces pancreatic juices
    c. There are two thyroid glands
3. State the passage of food from the mouth to the rectum.

References and Further Reading

Gregory, P. and Ward, A. (2010). *Sanders' Paramedic Textbook*. Edinburgh: Mosby Elsevier.

Hinson, J., Raven, P., and Chew, S. (2010). *The Endocrine System*, 2e. Edinburgh: Churchill Livingstone Elsevier.

Kleine, B. and Rossmanith, W.G. (2016). *Hormones and the Endocrine System: Textbook of Endocrinology*. London: Springer.

Peate, I. and Nair, M. (2016). *Fundamentals of Anatomy and Physiology: For Nursing and Healthcare Students*, 2e. Chichester: Wiley Blackwell.

Tortora, G.J. and Derrickson, B.H. (2017). *Tortora's Principles of Anatomy and Physiology*, 15e. Chichester: Wiley.

Waugh, A. and Grant, A. (2018). *Ross and Wilson Anatomy and Physiology*. Edinburgh: Elsevier.

The renal and urinary system

The renal and urinary system consists of the kidneys and the urinary bladder. It has many function within the body, these include

- Regulation of blood volume and pressure
- Regulation of the concentration of plasma ions
- Regulation of blood pH
- Conservation of nutrients

The kidneys

Lateral to the vertebrae and sit between the level of T12 and L3 in the Lumbar regions of the abdomen. They are retroperitoneal organs (sit behind the peritoneal sac) which means they may present with more localised pain if damaged or inflamed.

Renal capsule

- Fibrous covering of the kidney

Renal Cortex

- Functional part of the kidney (outer layer)

Medulla

- Middle section
- Contains 6–18 renal pyramids

Renal pyramids

- Functional units containing nephrons

Renal pelvis

- Concave area of kidneys where the ducts combine

Hilus (Hilum)

- Area where the *ureter* joins

Renal sinus

- Area where fluids enter

Nephron

- Glomerulus is the vascular capsule for filtration of the blood
- Bowmans capsule sits inside the Glomerulus for collection

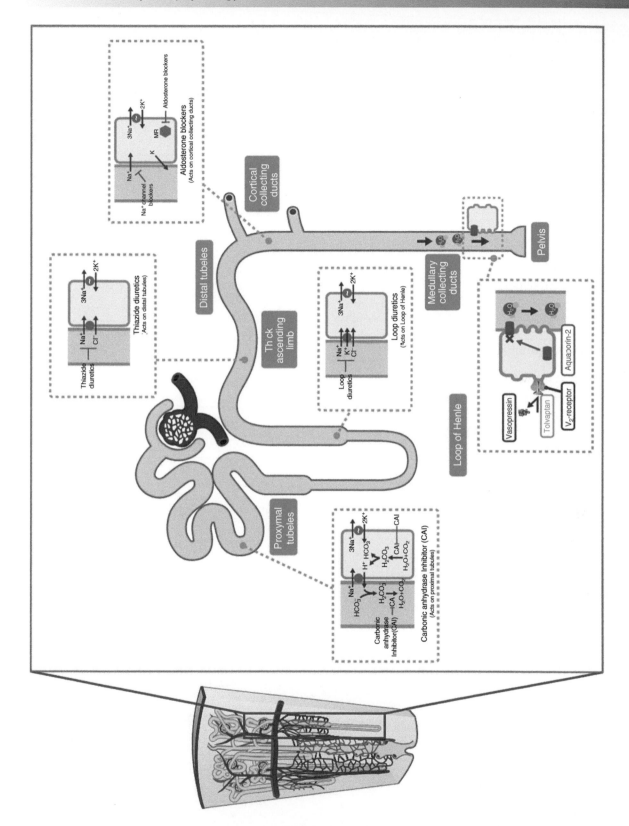

Figure 1.24   Labeled example of a nephron. Source: Mori et al. (2016). Diuretic usage for protection against end-organ damage in liver cirrhosis and heart failure. Hepatology Research, 47(1), 11–22.

Understanding what the nephrons does and how is important as patients can be on medication which affects areas of the nephrons. Also as a paramedic, you will have the ability to administer drugs that directly affect the nephrons.

The tubules

Proximal convoluted tubule

- Re-absorption of ions, organic molecules, vitamins and water
- These pass into interstitial spaces by diffusion

Descending loop of henle

- Re-absorption of water by osmosis

Ascending loop of henle

- Re-absorption of Cl^- and Na^+ increasing medullary concentration gradient

Distal convoluted tubule

- Selective re-absorption of Na^+ ions
- Secretion of amino acids and drugs

Transport mechanisms

Primary active transport

- Energy derived from 'hydrolysis' of ATP
- Substance actively 'pumped' across a membrane e.g. the sodium-potassium pump

Secondary active transport

- Uses proteins similar to facilitated diffusion
- Couples the movement of several separate substances in one cycle
- Utilises electrochemical gradients to drive the movement e.g. Na^+-Glucose transportation

Diuretic drugs

Loop diuretics

- *Decrease* Na^+ re-absorption through direct inhibition
- More fluid and solutes reach distal parts of renal tubule and get excreted

Thiazides

- Act on the distal convoluted tubule
- Promote loss of Na^+ and Cl^- to reduce re-absorption of fluid

Don't worry too much about these diuretic drugs at the moment; they will be covered in greater detail at level two. However, having a good basic understanding now will aid your practice.

Urinary

Ureters

- Transport fluid from kidneys to urinary bladder
- Approximately 25–35 cm long

Urinary bladder

- Temporary storage or urine for expulsion

Urethras

- Transport fluid from urinary bladder to the outside world

Questions

1. Fill in the blanks
   a. The kidneys sit between the level of _____ and _____
   b. The _____ transports fluid from the kidneys to the urinary bladder
   c. The renal hilum is where the _____ joins
2. Answer the following statements with true or false
   a. The renal cortex is the inner layer of the kidney
   b. The descending loop of henle re-absorbs water by osmosis
3. What does ATP stand for?
4. What are the four main functions of the renal system?
5. How many renal pyramids does the medulla contain?

References and Further Reading

Gregory, P. and Ward, A. (2010). *Sanders' Paramedic Textbook*. Edinburgh: Mosby Elsevier.

Peate, I. and Nair, M. (2016). *Fundamentals of Anatomy and Physiology: For Nursing and Healthcare Students*, 2e. Chichester: Wiley Blackwell.

Tarafdar, S. (2020). *Lecture Notes Nephrology: A Comprehensive Guide to Renal Medicine*. Chichester: Wiley Blackwell.

Tortora, G.J. and Derrickson, B.H. (2017). *Tortora's Principles of Anatomy and Physiology*, 15e. Chichester: Wiley.

Waugh, A. and Grant, A. (2018). *Ross and Wilson Anatomy and Physiology*. Edinburgh: Elsevier.

The skeletal system

Functions

- Support
- Protection
- Movement
- Mineral homeostasis
- Blood cell production
- Storage
  - Triclycerides stored as yellow bone marrow

Bone types

Long bones

- Major bones in the body e.g. femur

Short bones

- Smaller bones usually found in joints e.g. metacarpals in wrist

Flat

- Flat and thin bones e.g. skull

Irregular

- E.g. vertebrae

The skeleton can be separated into two distinct areas the Axial skeleton, which contains the skull, spine and ribs; and the Appendicular skeleton which contains everything else.

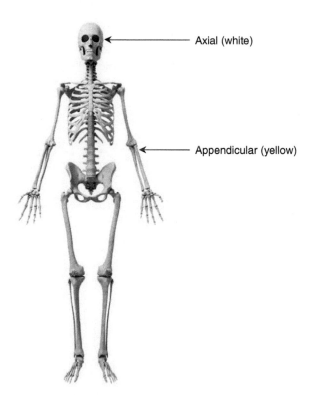

Axial (white)

Appendicular (yellow)

Figure 1.25 Representation of the axial and appendicular skeleton. Source: SciePro/Adobe Stock.

Joints

Within the body there are three main classifications of joints these are:
Fibrous

- Fixed immovable joints e.g. sutures of the skull

Cartilaginous

- Some degree of movement e.g. spine and ribs

Synovial

- Greater degree of movement e.g. knee
- Contains many structures within it

The spine

The spine is made up of **thirty-three** individual vertebrae they are separated into different sections of the spine.

Between the vertebrae, there are discs to allow for shock absorbance and movement. The spine has thirty-one pairs of spinal nerves.

Sections of the spine

- Cervical – 7 vertebrae
- Thoracic – 12 vertebrae
- Lumbar – 5 vertebrae
- Sacral – 5 fused vertebrae
- Coccyx – 4 fused vertebrae

Try to come up with a pneumonic to help you remember the sections of the spine and their order.

Spinal nerves

- Cervical – 8 pairs
- Thoracic – 12 pairs
- Lumbar – 5 pairs
- Sacral – 5 pairs
- Coccyx – 1 pair

References and Further Reading

Gregory, P. and Ward, A. (2010). *Sanders' Paramedic Textbook*. Edinburgh: Mosby Elsevier.
Nigg, B.M. and Herzog, W. (2007). *Biomechanics of the Musculo-skeletal System*. Chichester: Wiley.
Peate, I. and Nair, M. (2016). *Fundamentals of Anatomy and Physiology: For Nursing and Healthcare Students*, 2e. Chichester: Wiley Blackwell.
Tortora, G.J. and Derrickson, B.H. (2017). *Tortora's Principles of Anatomy and Physiology*, 15e. Chichester: Wiley.
Waugh, A. and Grant, A. (2018). *Ross and Wilson Anatomy and Physiology*. Edinburgh: Elsevier.

The muscular system

Functions

- Movement
- Body support and posture maintenance
- Heat production

Properties

Contractility

- Ability to shorten and change shape to become thicker

Excitability

- Capacity for fibres to respond to a stimuli

Extensibility

- Capacity to stretch beyond relaxed length

Elasticity

- Ability to return to original length after contracting or expanding

Muscle types

Cardiac

- Myocardium is innervated by Autonomic Nervous system
- Contractions are strong and rhythmic
- Myogenic (will continue to beat without stimuli)
- Anastomosing network (interlinked cells and fibres)

Smooth muscle

- Found in walls of hollow organs e.g. urinary bladder and uterus
- Found in walls of tubes e.g. respiratory, digestive, circulation
- Innervated by Autonomic Nervous system to regulate lumen size
- Contractions are strong and slow

Skeletal muscle

- Conscious control
- Approximately 40% of total body mass
- Contractions are rapid and forceful
- Structure
    - Endomysium surrounds each individual fibre
    - Perimysium surrounds fascicles (groups) of fibres
    - Epimysium surrounds the entire muscle

Anatomy

Tendons

- Bands of connective tissue binding muscle to bone
- Allow for movement across joints
- Supplied by sensory fibres that extend from muscular nerves

Ligaments

- Connective tissue across a binding bone to bone
- Easier to stretch than tendons
- Allow for a stable range of movement

Fascia

- Dense fibrous connective tissue forming bands or sheets
- Covers muscles, blood vessels and nerves
- Supports and anchors organs to nearby structures

Bursae

- Flattened sacs of synovial fluid
- Found where tendons rub against bones, ligaments or other tendons
- Prone to inflammation known as bursitis

Cartilage

- Connective tissue in joints etc.
- Acts as a surface for articulation
- Allows for smooth movement with reduced friction

References and Further Reading

Gregory, P. and Ward, A. (2010). *Sanders' Paramedic Textbook*. Edinburgh: Mosby Elsevier.

Nigg, B.M. and Herzog, W. (2007). *Biomechanics of the Musculo-skeletal System*. Chichester: Wiley.

Peate, I. and Nair, M. (2016). *Fundamentals of Anatomy and Physiology: For Nursing and Healthcare Students*, 2e. Chichester: Wiley Blackwell.

Tortora, G.J. and Derrickson, B.H. (2017). *Tortora's Principles of Anatomy and Physiology*, 15e. Chichester: Wiley.

Waugh, A. and Grant, A. (2018). *Ross and Wilson Anatomy and Physiology*. Edinburgh: Elsevier.

The integumentary system

The integumentary system represents the skin, hair, nails and accessory structures; including the sebaceous (oil) glands and the sudariferous (sweat) glands.

Functions

Protection

- Fluid loss
- Chemicals
- Physical trauma

- Bacteria
- Viruses
- Involuntary reflexes

Temperature maintenance

- Evaporation
- Conduction
- Convection

Storage of nutrients

- And production of Vitamin D

Sensory reception

- Many nerve endings in dermis

Excretion and secretion

- NaCl in sweat
- Other salts of substances e.g. garlic

Skin

The skin has three layers: the Epidermis, Dermis and the Subcutaneous or hypodermis.
   Epidermis

- Avascular, the nutrients are supplied by interstitial fluid
- No specialised nerve cells
- Contains many other structures
    - Openings of sweat glands
    - Melanocytes
    - Langerhans cells

Dermis

- Composed mainly of connective tissue containing collagen and elastin fibres
- Houses the glands of the skin
- Markel cells (sensory receptors)
- Defence cells (Hair follicles, fibroplasts, macrophages and mast cells)
- Blood vessels (Capillaries)

Subcutaneous (Hypodermis)

- Stabilising layer of the skin
- Largely made up of fat or loose connective tissue
- Contains arterioles and venules
- Insulating layer consisting of adipose tissue

Skin colour

The skin colour is dependent on two main chemicals Carotene and Melanin. Melanocyctes respond to Ultra-Violet light by producing melanin to protect the skin.

Aging

With age stem cell activity in the skin become reduced leading to a thinning of the skin and a greater sensitivity to sunlight. The skin will lose its elasticity with age and its ability to lose heat will diminish. The hair will also become thinner and change colour. Also with age would repair will take longer.

Wound repair

Many factors also have an impact on the body's ability to repair a wound.

Table 1.7   Components affecting wound repair.

Factor affecting wound repair	Complication
Nutrition	Wound healing requires a number of nutritional factors which may be missing in a poor diet
Diabetes	Reduction in vascularity Prone to infection due to high blood sugar levels
Renal disease	Fluid and electrolyte imbalance reduce cellular efficiency
Steroids (medication)	Inhibit the production of collagen needed for would repair
Age	Reduced cardiovascular function and tissue perfusion
Other factors	Foreign body in wound, infection, obesity, stress, location of wound i.e. highly mobile area?

Stages

1. Haemostasis
2. Inflammatory
3. Proliferative
4. Re-modelling

Haemostasis

- Vessel constriction
- Coagulation
- Clot formation

Inflammatory phase

- Begins at time of injury
- Clotting process

- Migration of fluid and other substances to affected area
- Ingestion of bacteria and debris
- Production of growth factors for next stage

Proliferative phase

- Building of new tissue to fill the wound space
- Fibroplasts synthesise and secrete collagen
- Protoglycans and glycoproteins required for would repair
- Epithelialisation

Re-modelling phase

- Approximately three weeks to six months after injury
- Decreased vascularity
- Re-modelling of scar tissue

The exact science of wound repair is definitely a nice to know at this stage it is covered more on Practitioner courses and by Doctors. Understanding that there are four stages involved and a basic knowledge of what each stage involves should be sufficient.

Questions

1. Fill in the blanks
   a. The radius is an example of a _____ bone
   b. The spine has _____ sections
   c. The three layers of the skin are _____, _____ and _____.
2. Answer the following statements with True or False
   a. A fibrous joint is freely movable
   b. The cervical spine has seven vertebrae
   c. Cardiac muscle contractions are rapid and forceful
   d. Ligaments binds bone to bone
3. What are the functions of the skeleton?
4. Define muscular excitability
5. How does the skin regulate temperature?
6. What effect does aging have on the skin?

References and Further Reading

Flanagan, M. (2013). *Wound Healing and Skin Integrity: Principles and Practice*. Chichester: Wiley Blackwell.

Gawkrodger, D. and Ardern-Jones, M.R. (2016). *Dermatology*, 6e. London: Elsevier.

Gregory, P. and Ward, A. (2010). *Sanders' Paramedic Textbook*. Edinburgh: Mosby Elsevier.

Peate, I. and Nair, M. (2016). *Fundamentals of Anatomy and Physiology: For Nursing and Healthcare Students*, 2e. Chichester: Wiley Blackwell.

Tortora, G.J. and Derrickson, B.H. (2017). *Tortora's Principles of Anatomy and Physiology*, 15e. Chichester: Wiley.
Waugh, A. and Grant, A. (2018). *Ross and Wilson Anatomy and Physiology*. Edinburgh: Elsevier.

Paediatrics

Paramedics are often more nervous when treating Paediatrics over any other group of patients. There are a few anatomical and physiological differences that are worth noting as it may effect your assessment and management. The main thing to remember is whilst they may not be 'just small adults' they are 'small humans'. Remembering this will take a lot of the stress out of treating them. If you think in terms of smaller physiology a lot of the differences will make sense.

Differences between adults and children

Childs airway

- Large head with short neck causing inability to support head
- Large occipital bone which means should be placed in neutral position to open airway
- Proportionally larger tongue creates a potential for obstruction
- Floor of mouth is easily compressible so hand placement during ventilation should be considered
- Infants under six months are obligate nasal breathers and prone to blockage
- Smaller diameter airways requiring less swelling to obstruct
- Epiglottis is horseshoe shaped and typically projects at 45°
- Larynx is usually high and anterior
- Trachea is short and soft with underdeveloped cartilage prone to oedema
- Cricoid ring is the smallest part compared to the Rima-glottis in an adult meaning an obstruction may be lower down
- Softer hard palate necessitating placement of oropharangeal airways to be anatomically (i.e. no turning)

Childs breathing

- Infants rely mainly on diaphragmatic breathing which can become obstructed by abdominal distension
- Ribs lie more horizontal contributing to a reduced chest expansion
- Muscles are more likely to fatigue than an adults
- Sternum and ribs are cartilaginous so may recess in severe respiratory distress
- Intercostal muscles are poorly developed leading to reduced chest compliance
- Increased metabolic rate so there is an increased oxygen demand
- Less elastic and collagen fibres in lungs increases chance of pulmonary oedema

Childs circulation

- Circulating volume is a greater proportion of total body weight
- Stroke volume is relatively fixed so a child can only compensate by increasing their heart rate
- Systemic vascular resistance rises after birth
- Unable to regulate temperature efficiently

Knowing these differences is useful to your practice as it helps you understand how a child may compensate and the differences of managing a young patient

References and Further Reading

Adewale, L. (2009). Anatomy and assessment of the paediatric airway. *Paediatric Anaesthesia* **19** (supp 1): 1–8.

Gregory, P. and Ward, A. (2010). *Sanders' Paramedic Textbook*. Edinburgh: Mosby Elsevier.

Lissauer, T. and Carroll, W. (2017). *Illustrated Textbook of Paediatrics*, 5e. London: Elsevier.

Peate, I. and Gormley-Fleming, E. (2015). *Fundamentals of Children's Anatomy and Physiology: A Textbook for Nursing and Healthcare Students*. Chichester: Wiley Blackwell.

Peate, I. and Nair, M. (2016). *Fundamentals of Anatomy and Physiology: For Nursing and Healthcare Students*, 2e. Chichester: Wiley Blackwell.

Tortora, G.J. and Derrickson, B.H. (2017). *Tortora's Principles of Anatomy and Physiology*, 15e. Chichester: Wiley.

Waugh, A. and Grant, A. (2018). *Ross and Wilson Anatomy and Physiology*. Edinburgh: Elsevier.

Practical skills for paramedics – 1

Contents

Being a Paramedic is a very hands-on and practical job; however, the most important practical skills are the so-called 'soft-skills'. These will allow you to interpret a scene and work quickly and effectively with other clinicians, emergency services and even the public.

The term 'Crew Resource Management' (CRM) encompasses how well you interact with others and utilise each other's skills to achieve a positive outcome, this is also in avoiding conflict that may jeopardise safety. Often people will use aviation analogies to demonstrate the principle of CRM, and there is one major limitation to applying this to healthcare – if a pilot makes an error, they are directly involved in the consequences. This is not the case, on the whole, for clinicians. Focussing on the aspects of care that will keep you safe as the rescuer will also protect your patients.

There are of course hands-on practical skills you will need to master throughout your training. These will be covered in this section and the following sections.

The Paramedic Revision Guide, First Edition. David W. Thom.
© 2021 John Wiley & Sons Ltd. Published 2021 by John Wiley & Sons Ltd.

Scene survey

When approaching a scene, you must first assess the scene before you can begin to start treating your patient or patients. When entering a scene, you must assess the dangers posed to:

- Yourself! Above all, you are the priority at all times
- Your crewmate. Always be conscious of danger posed to colleagues as they will also be looking out for you
- Public. Always ensure no further danger is posed to the public
- Patient. Notice the patient is last in line to be assessed for any danger posed to them, also be wary of any danger that may be posed by the patient

Danger can take many forms. So always assess the scene properly; don't be tempted to rush into the scene even if there are members of the public pulling you towards a patient. A risk assessment should always be dynamic, which means you should constantly reassess the scene as dangers may develop or become more prevalent. A dynamic risk assessment is especially important when you are dealing with a road traffic collision as the dangers may also include other services such as the fire service and their hydraulic equipment. Danger can be posed by (not exhaustive):

- Animals
- Public
- Traffic
- Fuel leaks
- Unstable structures
- Sharps
- Patients
- The list goes on just remember to **be careful**.

Always remember: *If in doubt, get out!*

Once you have assessed the scene and you have decided, it is safe you may then move onto treating your patient.

Remember DR. ABCDE

The initial assessment

On the first approach to a patient, you should always adopt a stepwise approach to ensure that you do not miss anything. With every patient, you should follow the following system.

Danger   (**DO I NEED HELP?**)

- Is the scene safe to approach? Use the previous page as a guide

Eyeball   (**DO I NEED HELP?**)

- This should be done during your scene survey so is not its own section
- Visually check for the pallor of the patient, are they pale or flushed? Are they clammy or diaphoretic (sweaty)? Are they cyanosed?
- Are they moving? Are they alert? Is there any respiratory effort? Are they talking?

Catastrophic haemorrhage <c>   (**DO I NEED HELP?**)

- Is there any sign of catastrophic haemorrhage? Is there an extenuating wound?
- This may have to be dealt with before other factors.

Response   (**DO I NEED HELP?**)

- Is the patient responding? For this, you should follow the AVPU structure step by step as once you have moved down the scale you cannot come back up
- A = Alert, is the patient alert and orientated?
- V = Voice, if they are not alert, do they respond to verbal stimuli

- P = Pain, if they do not respond to verbal stimuli, do they respond to a pain stimuli
  - Note that sternum rubs are not an acceptable form of pain stimuli use a trapezium squeeze instead
- U = Unresponsive, if they do not respond to any stimuli they are classified as unresponsive

C-spine <c>　　　　　　　　　　　　　　　　　　　　　　　　　　　　　**(DO I NEED HELP?)**

- Is there any evidence or trauma to suggest an injury to the C-spine
- Fall from a height? Head injury? Falling debris?

Airway　　　　　　　　　　　　　　　　　　　　　　　　　　　　　　**(DO I NEED HELP?)**

- Check the airway for any obstruction
- Remove any visible obstruction (remember to wear PPE!)
- Open the airway using a head tilt chin lift or jaw thrust if needed

Breathing　　　　　　　　　　　　　　　　　　　　　　　　　　　　　**(DO I NEED HELP?)**

- Check for respiratory effort
- Check an approximate rate, is it fast or slow?
- Are there any abnormal sounds?

Circulation　　　　　　　　　　　　　　　　　　　　　　　　　　　　**(DO I NEED HELP?)**

- Have they got a pulse?
- Is it fast or slow? Is it a strong pulse? Radial pulses? Bilateral pulses?

Disability　　　　　　　　　　　　　　　　　　　　　　　　　　　　　**(DO I NEED HELP?)**

- Are they awake?
- What is their blood sugar?

Exposure　　　　　　　　　　　　　　　　　　　　　　　　　　　　　**(DO I NEED HELP?)**

- What injuries do they have?
- What is their medical problem?
- What is their temperature?

> At all times think – **DO I NEED HELP**? The earlier you recognise a critically sick or injured patient, the earlier a critical care team can be involved. They are **NOT** just for trauma!

Unconsciousness

There are many causes for a patient to become unconscious. A handy pneumonic is **CHIEF SAP HEAD**.

- Cardiac
- Head injury
- Infantile convulsions
- Epilepsy
- Faint (syncope)

- Shock
- Anaphylaxis
- Poisoning

- Heat extremes
- Electrocution
- Apoploxy (stroke/CVA)
- Diabetes

> Cardiac arrest will be discussed later

Quick Questions

1. When entering a scene, what is the first thought?
2. What does AVPU stand for?
3. Who is the main priority at the scene?

References and Further Reading

Greaves, I. and Porter, K. (2007). *Oxford Handbook of Pre-Hospital Care*. Oxford: Oxford University Press.

Gregory, P. and Mursell, I. (2010). *Manual of Clinical Paramedic Procedures*. Chichester: Wiley Blackwell.

Gregory, P. and Ward, A. (2010). *Sanders' Paramedic Textbook*. Edinburgh: Mosby Elsevier.

Pilbery, R. and Lethbridge, K. (2019). *Ambulance Care Practice*, 2e. Bridgewater: Class Professional Publishing.

Royal College of Surgeons of Edinburgh (2019). *Generic Core Material: Prehospital Emergency Care Course*. Edinburgh: Royal College of Surgeons of Edinburgh.

Willis, S. and Dalrymple, R. (2020). *Fundamentals of Paramedic Practice: A Systems Approach*, 2e. Oxford: Wiley Blackwell.

Bleeding

> These patients need rapid intervention but their ongoing management may require a critical care team. Remember to recognise and call for help early.

During your career as a Paramedic, you will encounter a wide variety of bleeding. The most concerning one is catastrophic haemorrhage. Catastrophic haemorrhage, by its very definition, will result in the rapid and terminal exsanguination unless intervened upon.

Treatments for bleeding might include:

Pressure (direct and indirect)

- In the absence of readily available equipment, it may be required to apply pressure using your own body weight or grip
- More distal and superficial injures may be stemmed by this.

Tourniquets

- These should be applied early
- May require two to stem the bleeding
- Bony injuries may still ooze from the marrow

Pressure bandages

- A range of pressure bandages are available which may be useful

Remember to think that if you can see blood then there is likely more blood being lost that you cannot. It can be soaked into the surrounding area or being lost internally. Excessive amounts of blood that is lost should be replaced; most critical care teams in the UK carry blood or blood products to help with this.

References and Further Reading

Greaves, I. and Porter, K. (2007). *Oxford Handbook of Pre-Hospital Care*. Oxford: Oxford University Press.

Gregory, P. and Ward, A. (2010). *Sanders' Paramedic Textbook*. Edinburgh: Mosby Elsevier.

Royal College of Surgeons of Edinburgh (2019). *Generic Core Material: Prehospital Emergency Care Course*. Edinburgh: Royal College of Surgeons of Edinburgh.

Airway

The ultimate goal of the pre-hospital practitioner, for this section, is to ensure the patient has a patent airway and therefore is able to oxygenate. The appropriate intervention at the appropriate time for the patient is the correct approach. Try thinking about just because you have a hammer in the toolbox doesn't mean it is the right tool to remove a screw from the wall – even if it might indeed work one-way or another.

One overarching motto surrounds airway management: Do the basics first and do the basics well.

The majority of patients can be managed with simple manoeuvres and adjuncts for almost all situations. Of course, there are exceptions but by working hard to get the basics right, you will avoid having to perform more advanced procedures when they are not required.

You will never be judged for managing a patient on a simple adjunct and manoeuvre as long as that was sufficient to provide the patient with a patent airway and enable them to oxygenate.

Early recognition of complications is important, and this should be escalated appropriately to the suitable person, the earlier you call for a critical care team, the sooner they will be there. In the mean time, simple options will optimise the patient so that the critical care team are presented with a much more suitable patient.

Simple manoeuvres

Jaw thrust (Figure 2.1)

- Often underrated
- Simple
- Can be done with neck injuries
- Quick
- Beware of mandibular or facial injuries

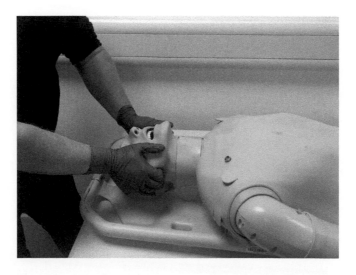

Figure 2.1   Jaw thrust.

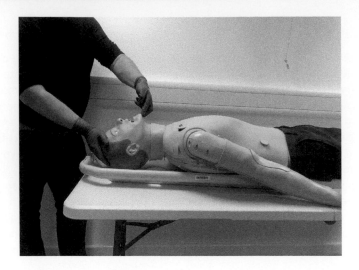

Figure 2.2   Head-tilt/Chin-lift.

Head tilt/chin lift (Figure 2.2)

- Quick
- Simple
- Effective
- Beware of the neck or spinal injuries

Airway positioning

Sniffing the morning air position (Figure 2.3)

- Does require pillow or similar
- Useful in optimising position

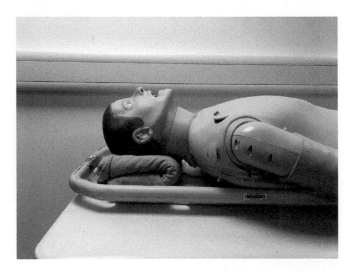

Figure 2.3   Sniffing the morning air position.

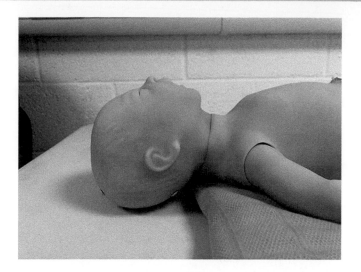

Figure 2.4 Neutral position for paediatric.

Paediatrics (Figure 2.4)

- Neutral position may be achieved by placing a blanket under the shoulders

  Ramping for obesity or pregnancy

- Optimises the airway position
- If the patient requires more intervention, they are in a good position
- If you pre-empt a difficult airway, it won't be a surprise
- Tragus of ear should be in line with sternum

All these techniques can be used in conjunction with simple adjuncts for extremely effective airway management

The majority of the time this will be all that the patient needs, if anything.

Simple adjuncts

Oropharyngeal airway (OPA)

- Inserted into the mouth of patients to aid in separation of tongue from soft palate
- Provides a tube for air passage through mouth
- Measured from the angle of the jaw to the flat plane of the incisors
- Inserted, in adults, backwards and then twisted in the mouth before advancing to aid in the movement of the tongue
- Contraindicated in patients with a gag reflex

Nasopharyngeal Airway (NPA)

- Adjunct of choice in trismus (clenched jaw)
- Inserted perpendicular to the face into nose with the bevel to the septum
  - Do **NOT** angle the NPA as it will hit the bones in the nose and may cause damage. By pointing directly to back of the patients' head, it should go in without resistance.

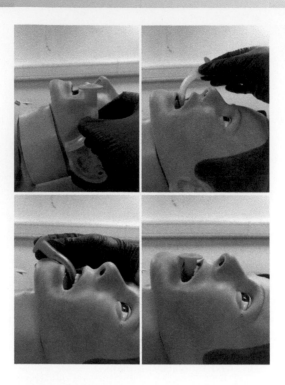

Figure 2.5 OPA insertion.

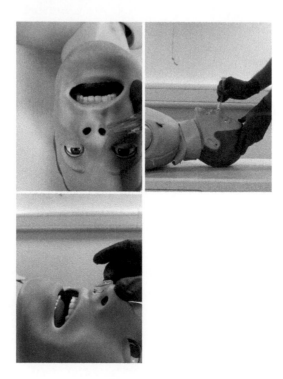

Figure 2.6 NPA insertion.

- Requires lubrication
- Can cause bleeding
- May be tolerated more easily in patients with a higher level of consciousness than an OPA
- Measured from the tragus of the ear to the tip of the nose
- Cautioned in patients with suspected basal skull fractures
- Do not continue to insert if resistance is met

Supraglottic Airway Devices (SAD)

Two main types used in the UK are the iGel™ and Laryngeal Mask Airway devices
  Laryngeal Mask Airway (LMA)

- Reduces the risk of aspiration compared with OPA's but does not prevent
- Size determined by the weight of a patient
- Check it inflates and holds air before inserting
- 'Cowboy hat' shape
- Hold like a pen and inserted anatomically along the hard and soft palate with the head in the 'sniffing the morning air' position
- Release when inflating
- The maximum volume of air to inflate is: (SIze of LMA $-1) \times 10 =$ mL of air
    - E.g. a size 4 LMA is $(4-1) \times 10 = 30$ mL of air. But remember this is a maximum and may not need all to get a seal.

  iGel™

- Creates a better seal than traditional LMA's
- Moulds to the patients' airway
- Does not require inflation
- Inserted similarly.

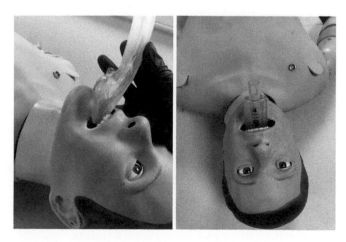

Figure 2.7   iGel insertion.

Bag-Valve-Mask (BVM)

- The BVM provides **positive pressure** ventilation to patients.
- Three main sizes
  - Adult
  - Paediatric
  - Neonatal
- The bag is larger than the lung capacity of most patients so don't squeeze it all
- May worsen a pneumothorax by providing positive pressure if untreated
- The patients face should be drawn into the mask **NOT** the mask pushed onto their face.
- Works with simple airway manoeuvres and adjuncts

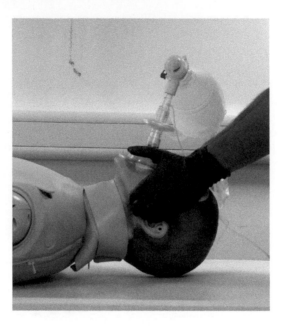

Figure 2.8   Two-handed technique with BVM.

Choking

When patient is choking, it is vital to recognise the symptoms as quickly as possible as quick intervention will save your patient.

Mild cases (with effective cough)

- Encourage coughing to assist in the movement of the blockage

Severe cases (ineffective cough)

- Administer five back blows
- If back blows are ineffective then administer five abdominal thrusts
  - Note if you have administered abdominal thrusts to a patient then they must attend hospital due to the risk of internal injuries
  - Children under one should receive chest thrusts
- If the blockage persists recommence cycle with five back blows
- If your patients become unconscious begin Cardiopulmonary Resuscitation (CPR) immediately

It's worth reviewing the Resuscitation Council guidelines for choking at this point!

Beginning CPR is a common practice to forget so it's well worth understanding early on! Once CPR has begun you are essentially providing chest thrusts to the patient to remove the blockage

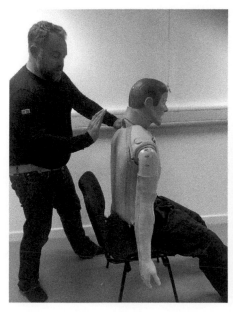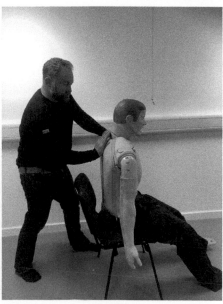

Figure 2.9   Back blows.

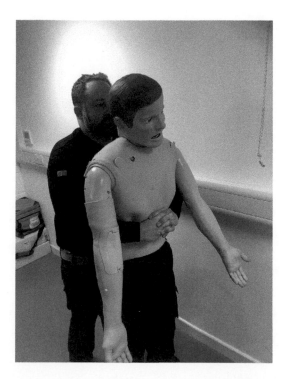

Figure 2.10   Abdominal thrusts.

Quick Questions

1. Why do children require a neutral head position when opening an airway?
2. What is the maximum volume of air you would use to inflate a size 5 LMA?
3. How do you size an NPA?
4. Is fine VF a shockable rhythm?
5. What checks should you make before attaching the pads to a patient?

References and Further Reading

Difficult Airway Society (2015). DAS guidelines for management of unanticipated difficult intubation in adults 2015. https://das.uk.com/guidelines/das_intubation_guidelines (accessed 30 October 2020).

Greaves, I. and Porter, K. (2007). *Oxford Handbook of Pre-Hospital Care*. Oxford: Oxford University Press.

Gregory, P. and Mursell, I. (2010). *Manual of Clinical Paramedic Procedures*. Chichester: Wiley Blackwell.

Gregory, P. and Ward, A. (2010). *Sanders' Paramedic Textbook*. Edinburgh: Mosby Elsevier.

Hammond, B.B. and Zimmermann, P.G. (2013). *Sheehy's Manual of Emergency Care*, 7e. Missouri: Mosby.

Pilbery, R. and Lethbridge, K. (2019). *Ambulance Care Practice*, 2e. Bridgewater: Class Professional Publishing.

Pino, R.M. (2015). *Clinical Anesthesia Procedures of the Massachusetts General Hospital*, 9e. Philadelphia: Wolters Kluwer.

Resuscitation Council UK (2015). Choking. https://www.resus.org.uk/choking/ (accessed 30 October 2020).

Royal College of Surgeons of Edinburgh (2019). *Generic Core Material: Prehospital Emergency Care Course*. Edinburgh: Royal College of Surgeons of Edinburgh.

Willis, S. and Dalrymple, R. (2020). *Fundamentals of Paramedic Practice: A Systems Approach*, 2e. Oxford: Wiley Blackwell.

Yezid, N.H., Poh, K., Md Noor, J. et al. (2019). *BMJ Case Reports CP* **12**: e230201. https://doi.org/10.1136/bcr-2019-230201.

Basic life support and defibrillation

Basic life support (BLS) is the maintenance of airway patency, support mechanisms of breathing and circulation without the use of equipment. At level one, you will undertake a modified form of basic life support as you should be competent in basic airway adjuncts, the use of a bag valve mask (BVM) and a defibrillator.

Adults

Before beginning BLS, you must first assess the patients need for the procedure. This is done using the primary survey that was discussed earlier.

1. D<c>R<c>ABC
   Confirmed cardiac arrest?
   a. No effort of breathing no pulse? (agonal is counted as lack of respiratory effort)

   Stepwise approach

- Danger
  - Assess the scene
- Eyeball
  - Remember to consider any catastrophic haemorrhage or any evidence of C-spine
- Response
  - AVPU
- Airway
  - Is it clear? If not then clear it.
  - Open airway by head tilt chin or jaw thrust

> Agonal breathing can be hard to determine but if you are unsure of a pulse and the patients breathing is not 'normal' then consider it to be agonal. Gasps as well as rapid shallow breaths can be agonal.

- Breathing
  - Look, listen and feel for up to 10 seconds
- Circulation
  - Check carotid pulse for up to 10 seconds
  - This can be conducted at the same time as your breathing assessment
- No pulse, no breathing? Begin chest compressions and **call for help – get a second crew!**
  - In adults, the ratio is 30 : 2 at a rate of 100–120 per minutes
- Attach the defibrillator as early as possible (utilise a bystander to take over compressions if available)
  - Remember 5 P's (we will cover these later)
  - Assess rhythm. Shockable or non-shockable?
  - Remember to minimise time of the chest when assessing the rhythm
- Shockable? '**STAND CLEAR I AM GOING TO SHOCK' + Visual check**
  - Administer first shock as per the device you are using.
  - Minimise time off the chest.
  - Defibrillation checks (covered later)
- Non-shockable? Continue CPR
- Continue with CPR
  - Ratio of 30 : 2 using a BVM to ventilate
  - Place airway adjunct as soon as possible
  - After five cycles (or two minutes) reassess rhythm as treat appropriately.

> Time of the chest is crucial so keep it to a minimum

ROSC

If a Return Of Spontaneous Circulation (ROSC) occurs it is then vital to reassess your patients' needs as soon as possible. Once again you must follow the stepwise approach

Airway

- Is it still patent?
  - Remember providing chest compressions and the use of a BVM can cause emesis (vomiting) which may occlude the airway in addition to salivary build up
- If they have an adjunct in place, are they tolerating it still?
- Do they need suctioning?

Breathing

- Is the patient making any respiratory effort?
- What rate?
- Does it need assisting?

> Aim 10–12 assisted breaths per minute at this level. Later, we will discuss CO_2

Circulation

- Does the pulse correlate with what is shown on the monitor?
- Check for systemic circulation, do they have a radial? Is it strong, weak, bounding etc?
- Capillary refill time? Is it <two seconds?

The main priorities when conducting any resuscitation is to minimise the time off the chest and ensure high-quality chest compressions are achieved with early defibrillation! This is what will make the difference in survival for patients.

Reversible causes

When conducting BLS, you should have an awareness of the reversible causes of cardiac arrest. Some of which we can intervene and attempt to reverse, some we cannot at this stage.

Four H's

- Hypoxia
  - Reduced oxygen perfusion can cause fatal cardiac arrests. This is why it is important to ensure the airway is clear so that the oxygen being ventilated into a patient reached the lungs
- Hypothermia
  - Are they in a cold environment? What's their temperature?
- Hypovolaemia
  - Low levels of circulating blood can lead to cardiac arrest. At this level, there is not a lot you can do to treat this but be aware a patient can lose vast amounts of blood into the abdomen, pelvis and long bones
- Hypo/Hyperkalaemia (and other metabolic disorders)
  - Hypo/Hyperkalaemia refers to the levels of calcium in the blood, which can result in cardiac arrest. This is not a cause that can be reversed by the ambulance.
  - However, we can measure one metabolic disorder through checking the patient's blood sugar levels which may be reversible

Four T's

- Toxins
  - Look out for any signs of toxins this can be through track marks (which could be a reversible cause) dog bites, wounds and chemicals
- Thrombus
  - This is not one that can't usually be treated in the pre-hospital setting; however, the critical care team may carry thrombolytic drugs.
  - Look out for possible history which might suggest this
- Tamponade
  - This cannot be reversed by the ambulance staff and carries a high mortality rate. Typically, it will present with a Pulseless Electrical Activity (PEA)
- Tension Pneumothorax
  - This is manageable with skills in level two so be aware of the signs which include unequal chest expansion on ventilation and quiet breath sounds on auscultation
  - Remember this can be caused by you using positive pressure ventilation with the BVM

> The BLS algorithm and reversible causes should be learnt verbatim and ad nauseam.

Quick Questions

1. Why can Hypo/Hyperkalaemia cause cardiac arrest?
2. What are the two primary considerations when conducting BLS?
3. How do you confirm cardiac arrest?
4. What are the steps to BLS

Paediatric basic life support

This is an area that will be covered more in level two but there are some basics that it is definitely worth knowing

Classification

Newborn

- Just after birth

Neonate

- Fist 28 days of life

Infant

- Child under one year of age

Child

- From one year old to puberty

Paediatric basics

With a paediatric, you still follow the same D<c>R<c>ABC formula; however, after confirming cardiac arrest, the methodology is slightly different as in children the leading cause for cardiac arrest in hypoxia. Make sure to refer to local policy and procedures.

1. Open airway
    a. Head in require neutral position rather than chin lift
2. Not breathing?
3. Administer five rescue breaths (remember to use a BVM, not your mouth)
4. Reassess breathing and circulation
5. If still in cardiac arrest administer chest compressions with a ratio of 15 : 2
6. **Call for help from a critical care team early!**

Defibrillation

Defibrillation is the delivery of a direct current shock through the myocardium of the heart.

It works by *stopping* the heart to encourage it to restart in a normal rhythm.

It is the definitive treatment for Ventricular Fibrillation and *Pulseless* Ventricular Tachycardia so do not delay delivery of a shock!

When attaching the defibrillator, you must first check the 5 P's of defibrillation. These are used to assess the suitability of an area for pad placement.

Five P's

Expose the chest and assess for:

1. Pendants or Piercings (remove if possible or consider pad placement, remember these remain the property of the patient at all times)
2. Patches (these can be GTN, nicotine and other nitrates. Remove if possible or consider pads placement)
3. Pacemaker (never place the defibrillator pads over a pacemaker site)
4. Perspiration or other fluids (this can include drowned patients or patients lying on a wet floor. Dry patient first if possible and never defibrillate a patient in a pool of water!)
5. Playtex or underwire bra (remove if possible but remember the patients' dignity)

Rhythms

Shockable
Pulseless Ventricular Tachycardia (VT)

- Remember to always check for a pulse with this rhythm
- Heart is being innervated by an area other than the SA node

Ventricular Fibrillation (VF)

- Heart is being innervated by multiple points causing no controlled contraction

NON-shockable
Asystole

- Heart lacks electrical innervations
- CHECK LEADS! It could be due to a connection error

Pulseless Electrical Activity (PEA)

- Patient will have electrical activity in the heart, but the mechanical action of pumping will be affected
- This could be due to cardiac tamponade or other factors
- If it isn't VF, VT or asystole and <u>doesn't</u> have a pulse it is PEA. The exact rhythm is a moot point.

Defibrillation

When you are defibrillating a patient, there is a set structure so that nothing is missed this is for your safety as well as the patients.

1. Attach monitor whilst checking the 5 P's
2. Stop chest compressions to assess rhythm
3. First command 'VF/VT/PEA/Asystole seen! Confirm?'
   a. Confirming the rhythm with your colleague allows you to be confident in the treatment that follows
   b. Remember for VT and PEA you check a pulse!
   c. Remember for Asystole you check the leads
4. Shockable? Charge the defibrillator
   a. When the defibrillator charging continues with chest compressions!
5. Monitor fully charged? Stop chest compressions
6. Verbalise and check Top, middle and bottom. Using this sequence ensures no area is missed. Ask colleagues to move if they are in contact with the patient
7. 'Lines down. Oxygen away. Hands up'
   a. This ensures that no one is connected to the patient in anyway and the risks of igniting the oxygen is reduced
   b. The team raising their hands is a visual clue that no one is touching the patient
8. 'Stand clear'
9. Final visual check and deliver shock
10. Immediately recommence BLS
    a. In total, from stopping chest compressions to delivering, the shock the entire process should take no more than 10 seconds
    b. Do not stop to recheck a pulse after defibrillating, wait until the next rhythm check

> It might be worth revisiting the ECG page to look at rhythms at this point.

> This whole sequence should take a matter of seconds and absolutely no more than 10.

Reassess after five cycles of 30 : 2 or two minutes and administer subsequent shocks as required

Limiting factors

Many factors can limit the effectiveness of defibrillation

- Transthoracic impedance
  - Resistance to the flow of electricity
- Hairy chest
  - This will decrease the pad's contact with the skin
- Pad placement
  - Care should be taken to ensure the current would travel through the heart.
- Number of shocks
  - The pads will degrade with subsequent shocks, consider changing both pads and position after four to five shocks. This must not delay another shock though.

Pad placement

On an adult patient, you would always aim to place the pads in the anterior–anterior position. However, there may be times when this is not possible, consider the five P's, and therefore, anterior–posterior placement is available. On children, this may be the only available placement due to the size of the pads.

If defibrillation continually fails to terminate VF/VT in the anterior–anterior placement then you should change to the anterior–posterior placement or axillary.

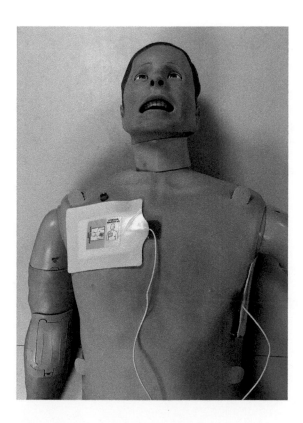

Figure 2.11   Anterior – anterior.

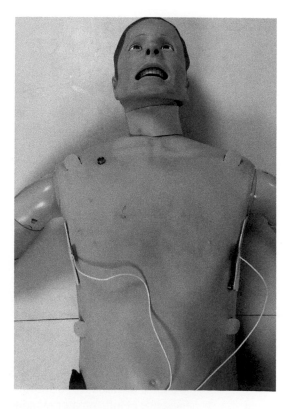

Figure 2.12   Axillary – axillary.

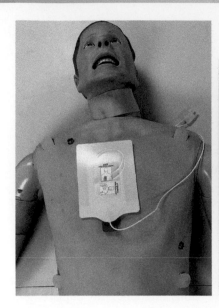 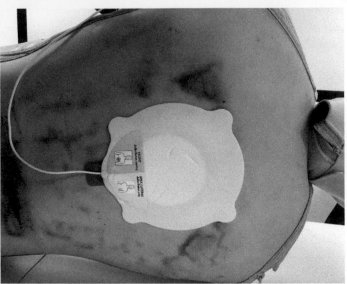

Figure 2.13   Anterior – posterior.

References and Further Reading

Greaves, I. and Porter, K. (2007). *Oxford Handbook of Pre-Hospital Care*. Oxford: Oxford University Press.

Gregory, P. and Mursell, I. (2010). *Manual of Clinical Paramedic Procedures*. Chichester: Wiley Blackwell.

Gregory, P. and Ward, A. (2010). *Sanders' Paramedic Textbook*. Edinburgh: Mosby Elsevier.

Hammond, B.B. and Zimmermann, P.G. (2013). *Sheehy's Manual of Emergency Care*, 7e. Missouri: Mosby.

Pilbery, R. and Lethbridge, K. (2019). *Ambulance Care Practice*, 2e. Bridgewater: Class Professional Publishing.

Resuscitation Council UK (2015). Adult basic life support and automated external defibrillation. https://www.resus.org.uk/resuscitation-guidelines/adult-basic-life-support-and-automated-external-defibrillation/ (accessed 30 October 2020).

Royal College of Surgeons of Edinburgh (2019). *Generic Core Material: Prehospital Emergency Care Course*. Edinburgh: Royal College of Surgeons of Edinburgh.

Willis, S. and Dalrymple, R. (2020). *Fundamentals of Paramedic Practice: A Systems Approach*, 2e. Oxford: Wiley Blackwell.

Shock

Types of shock

- Hypovolaemic
- Cardiogenic
    - Inability of the heart to fill or pump properly
- Obstructive
    - Obstruction of the outflow from the heart (i.e. pneumothorax, PE, tamponade)
- Distributive
    - Loss of vasomotor tone (i.e. neurogenic)
    - Presence of vasodilating substances in blood (i.e. anaphylaxis)
    - Presence of inflammatory mediators (i.e. septic)

Hypovolaemic

Caused by loss of blood or electrolytes

Compressible controllable haemorrhage

Non-compressible non-controllable haemorrhage

Open wounds which can be controlled by direct or indirect pressure. This can be assisted by wound packing, dressing or tourniquets

Major blood loss will occur if not treated as much as possible. Usually, internal injuries and predominantly caused by major trauma

Stages

	Stage 1 **15% (750 mL)**	**Stage 2** **15–30% (750–1500 mL)**	**Stage 3** **30–40% (1500–2000 mL)**	**Stage 4** **40%+** **(>2000 mL)**
Pulse	<100	100–120	120–140	140+
BP (systolic)	Normal	Normal	100 mmHg	90 mmHg
Pulse pressure	Normal	Falling+	Falling++	Falling+++
Respiratory rate	Normal	20–30	30–40	30–35
Skin	Pallor	Cold, clammy	Cold, clammy	Moribund
Capillary refill	Normal	Positive	Positive	Positive

Whilst this model is still taught, it is unhelpful in practice. Patient's may compensate for longer than stated or may present earlier. Medications such as beta-blockers may alter the physiological findings and render this table obsolete. Early recognition and management are the key here. Firstly, recognise they are in shock and then which type. Calling for help early from a pre-hospital critical care team might prove beneficial here.

Anaphylaxis

Anaphylaxis is a severe and potentially fatal form of a hypersensitivity reaction, which eventually affects all organs usually (but not always) evoked by an antigen.

The antigen results in the body releasing, amongst other things, histamine.

This causes constriction of smooth muscle in the lungs, dilatation of arterioles and capillaries whilst increasing the capillary permeability (Table 2.1).

Effects on each system:

Table 2.1 Effects of anaphylaxis on different systems.

Cardiac	Respiratory	Skin
Decreased coronary blood flow	Spasmodic oedema of bronchi	Urticaria
Reduced cardiac output	Pulmonary vasoconstriction	Pruritis
Systemic vasodilatation	Laryngeal oedema	Oedema
Increased blood vessel permeability		

Early symptoms of an allergic reaction include:

- Anxiety and lightheadedness
- Tingling
- Itching and urticaria
- Tongue swelling and eye irritation
- Warmth
- Nasal congestion and/or sneezing

Anaphylaxis

- Extreme dyspnoea
  - Wheezing, coughing, stridor, prolonged sneezing
- Tachycardia
  - Sometimes accompanied by arrhythmias
- Severe hypotension
  - Due to vasodilatation
- Warm flushed skin
  - Pallor as patient deteriorates
- Oedema
  - Particularly around face and airway
- Pruritis
  - Severe itching
- Nausea, vomiting and abdominal cramps

> The endogenous anti-dote for histamine is adrenaline. It is important to remember this when treating anaphylaxis

Cardiogenic

Causes

- Primary myocardial failure
- Arrhythmia
- Tamponade
- Tension pneumothorax
- Contusion
- Heart failure
- Reduction in cardiac output
  - Decreased blood supply
  - Decreased oxygen delivery

Assess your patient for signs of

- Heart failure
- Tamponade
  - Tachycardia
  - Muffled heart sounds
  - Engorged neck veins with hypotension
  - Dyspnoea
  - Oedema of feet and ankles
- Tension pneumothorax
- Cardiac dysrhythmia
- Myocardial infarction

Neurogenic

Caused by:

- Spinal cord injury
- Certain drugs
- Brainstem, spinal or torso trauma

Will usually occur between

- C1–C2
- C7
- T12–L1

Signs and symptoms

- Hypotension without tachycardia
- Low blood pressure with minimal response to fluids
- Venous pooling inferior to injury

Questions

1. Complete the table on the stages of hypovolaemic shock

	Stage 1 ___% (750 mL)	**Stage 2** 15–30% (750–1500 mL)	**Stage 3** 30–40% (_____-_____mL)	**Stage 4** 40%+ (>2000 mL)
Pulse	<100	____-____	120–140	140+
BP (systolic)	Normal	Normal	100 mmHg	___mmHg
_____ _____	Normal	Falling+	Falling++	Falling+++
Respiratory rate	Normal	20–30	___-___	30–35
Skin	Pallor	_____	Cold, clammy	Moribund
Capillary refill	_____	Positive	Positive	Positive

2. What is anaphylaxis?

References and Further Reading

Greaves, I. and Porter, K. (2007). *Oxford Handbook of Pre-Hospital Care*. Oxford: Oxford University Press.

Gregory, P. and Ward, A. (2010). *Sanders' Paramedic Textbook*. Edinburgh: Mosby Elsevier.

Hammond, B.B. and Zimmermann, P.G. (2013). *Sheehy's Manual of Emergency Care*, 7e. Missouri: Mosby.

Royal College of Surgeons of Edinburgh (2019). *Generic Core Material: Prehospital Emergency Care Course*. Edinburgh: Royal College of Surgeons of Edinburgh.

Wound classification

Contusion

- Caused by blunt trauma
- Blood vessels rupture to cause ecchymosis (bruising)
- Blood loss deeper in tissues is known as a Haematoma

Laceration

- Snagging, tearing or splitting of tissue
- Causes include barbed wire, machinery and broken glass
- Freely bleeding
- Prolonged healing time

Incision

- Caused by a sharp object or blade e.g. knife
- Linear wound
- Bleeds freely
- Relatively quick to heal

Puncture

- Caused by a sharp pointed injury
- Small entrance wound
- Potential for underlying injury
- Check for
    - Contamination
    - Retained foreign bodies
    - Associated injuries

Although these may not seem important now, they ensure a common language between the ambulance service and receiving clinicians in the hospital as well as for medico-legal cases

Abrasion

- Partial-thickness injury
- Caused by friction
- Removal of layer or layers of skin
- Painful due to nerve endings

Avulsion

- Full-thickness skin loss 'degloving'
- Wound edges cannot be approximated
- Causes include industrial equipment and bites
- Avulsed tissue may be salvageable

Bleeding

Bleeding can be divided into three types:
Arterial

- Bright red in colour (frank blood)
- Spurts in time with the pulse

Venous

- Dark red to purple in colour
- Continuous flow

Capillary

- 'Oozing'
- Common from abrasions

Treatment

1. Gloves!
   a. Be sure to wear PPE at all times when there is a risk of contamination by bodily fluid.
2. Expose wound
   a. This allows for a more in-depth examination
   b. Apply direct or indirect pressure to the wound or around embedded object
   c. Remember never to remove any embedded objects
4. Apply pressure
   a. Direct or indirect
2. Dress the wound
   a. Sterile dressings
2. Document and refer
   a. Make sure to document your findings and treatment

Indirect pressure is the application on pressure to an artery with the aim to reduce the blood loss from the wound distal to the pressure area.

Burns and scalds

Burns and scalds can be classified into six generic categories.
Dry burn

- Caused by flames or friction etc.

Scald

- Caused by steam or hot liquids

Electrical burn

- Low or high voltages can cause burns

Cold injury

- Frostbite or contact with freezing materials

Chemical burn

- Industrial and domestic chemicals have the ability to burn

Radiation burn

- Sunburn or a radioactive source

Remember patients are three dimensional so check the back as well!

Assessment

The approach to burns will follow the standard 'DR ABCDE' approach, but there are some specific things to look for with burns.

- Consider personal safety, if in doubt move away into a safe area
- Consider the time that has elapsed since the burn and any first aid that has been applied i.e. running under cool water
- Consider the source of the burn and type
- Determine the extent of the burn (size)
- Determine the location of the burn; does it affect the mouth, face or throat?
- Determine the depth of the burn

Burn sizing

The size of a burn is described in terms of a percentage of the total body surface area (%TBSA). This will guide treatment later. Often the size of the burn is over-sized pre-hospitally. There are a few ways to do this; Rule of Nines, Serial halving, Palm size and the Lund and Browder chart. There are also mobile phone apps available to help.

Erythema (redness) is **NOT** included in the burn size. Only the areas that are actually burnt.

Rule of Nines

- The body is split into segments
- Each section is assigned a percentage
- If the area is fully burnt then add that number to the %TBSA
- Drawbacks are as follows: it is difficult to remember and, unless the section is fully burnt, it is hard to assess

Serial Halving

- Divide the body into half sections (vertically)
- If the burn is smaller than that then divide horizontally
- Repeat these steps until a number is reached that represents the burnt area
- Useful for larger burns

- Quick
- Not particularly accurate

Palm size

- Using *the patients'* hand as a guide to estimate burns
- The whole hand *including* the digits is approximately 0.8% of the total body surface area
- This is typically described as 1% but will overestimate the burn size
- May be uncomfortable or painful
- Useful for smaller and distal burns
- Can use a rough template on some paper for the size

> **MUST** be the whole hand **INCLUDING** the digits for the size.

Lund and Browder chart

- Most accurate method
- Requires the chart (although mobile phone apps are available)
- More time-consuming in the pre-hospital environment therefore may be more beneficial to try another method.

Considerations

- Airway burns are dangerous as they may cause swelling and close the airway
- Full-thickness burn should be treated in specialist centres
- Circumferential burns to torso or limbs may require pre-hospital surgical input
- Partial-thickness burns larger than 1% may require specialist support
- Superficial burns larger than 5% may require specialist input

> 1% TBSA is much bigger than you might think. Try putting your palm (including digits) on your stomach and add a bit more to get an idea.

Classification

Superficial

- Affects the epidermis but not the dermis e.g. sunburn
- Erythema (redness) present and potential for blistering
- Rapid healing, usually within one week

Partial-thickness

- Affects upper dermis and the epidermis
- Exposed nerve ending make the wound very painful
- Blistering and paleness
- Healing usually occurs within two weeks

Full thickness

- Notoriously difficult to assess
- Non-blanching
- Bleeding is delayed due to damaged vessels
- Often less painful than partial-thickness due to damages nerve endings
- Healing can take weeks to months due to damaged regeneration of cells
- Appear dry and waxy or leathery

Treatment

1. Remove source if it is safe to do so
   a. This may mean removing patient from scene
2. Cool the burn with cool fresh water for a minimum 20 minutes
   a. If it is a chemical burn then cool for a minimum of an hour (this can be done on the way to hospital after initial cooling.
3. Remove patients' rings, watches, belts etc if on or near affected area
   a. Always return property to the patient do not keep hold of it
4. Never peel adhered clothing
5. Provide analgesia
   a. Cooling will help with the pain as well as analgesics
6. Cover with a sterile dressing and/or cling film
   a. Ensure to use strips of cling film lengthways, never wrap the wound as it may inhibit expansion of tissues due to inflammation
   b. By stopping the air getting to the burn, it will reduce the pain
7. Consider the need for assistance from critical care teams
8. Involve the local burn care network and follow their guidance on destination

Quick Questions

1. What is ecchymosis?
2. How would you describe venous bleeding?
3. When would you apply indirect pressure?
4. Degloving is more formally known as?
5. How would you estimate the extent of a burn?
6. How would you classify a superficial burn?

References and Further Reading

Greaves, I. and Porter, K. (2007). *Oxford Handbook of Pre-Hospital Care*. Oxford: Oxford University Press.

Gregory, P. and Ward, A. (2010). *Sanders' Paramedic Textbook*. Edinburgh: Mosby Elsevier.

Hammond, B.B. and Zimmermann, P.G. (2013). *Sheehy's Manual of Emergency Care*, 7e. Missouri: Mosby.

Royal College of Surgeons of Edinburgh (2019). *Generic Core Material: Prehospital Emergency Care Course*. Edinburgh: Royal College of Surgeons of Edinburgh.

Thom, D. (2017). Appraising current methods for preclinical calculation of burn size - a pre-hospital perspective. *Burns* **43** (1): 127–136.

Fractures and dislocations

Definitions

Fracture

- A break in the continuity of a bone. This can be complete fracture or incomplete

Dislocation

- The displacement of one or more bones at a joint

Sprain

- The over stretching and/or tearing of a *ligament* at a joint

Strain

- The over stretching and/or tearing of a muscle

Fracture classification

Closed

- Skin and soft tissues surrounding the fracture are still intact
- No direct contamination
- Significant blood loss can still occur

Open

- Overlying wound to the fracture causing the bone to be exposed
- May be caused by a penetrating injury or by the bone itself
- High risk of infection (osteomyelitis)
- Can lose more blood than a closed fracture

Signs and symptoms

Tenderness	Deformity	Haematoma
Crepitus	Swelling	Haemorrhage
Unnatural movement	Shortening	Rotation
Absent distal pulses	Absent or reduced sensation	Ischemia or poor perfusion

Compartment syndrome

A small risk with any fracture is the development of compartment syndrome, which is where the haemorrhage from the fracture is trapped within the facia of the muscles leading to an increased pressure. This can present with extreme pain, paraesthesia (pins and needles), pallor, and a lack of pulse.

Dislocations

Dislocation

- Separation of two bones at a joint
- Result of severe disruption to the ligaments
- Patients with previous dislocations have a higher risk or reoccurrence
- Threatens neurovascular status of the limb
- Normally presents with obvious deformity and pain at a joint

Facture dislocation

- Difficult to differentiate from a fracture
- Severe damage caused to underlying structure
- Carries a huge risk of neurovascular compromise
- Doctors may reduce on scene if present

Paediatrics

Fractures and dislocations in children can be very difficult to identify and children are notoriously difficult to assess especially when they are distressed or in pain.

- Be aware of the mechanism of injury as this may give you a better idea
- Remember a greater force is required to fracture children's bones
- Does the story add up? Are there other injuries?
    - First step in identifying non-accidental injury is thinking about it in the first place
- Epiphyseal fractures occur when a growth plate becomes dislodged
- Usually receive greenstick fractures to the bones having a greater flexibility

Pre-hospital management

- Create a safe working environment (especially if caused by external forces)
- Control external haemorrhage
- Reduce pain (this may be mechanical or pharmacological)
- Expose and examine (look, feel, move)
- Prevent further injury (immobilisation of injury)
- Ensure neurovascular supply distal to the injury (may require reduction by a suitably trained clinician – consider the critical care team)
- Remove jewellery distal to the injury
- Regularly reassess wound and patient
- Transport to definitive care
- If the fracture is open (i.e. bone is showing) then consider antibiotics
    - An open fracture is one where the bone has pierced out through the skin, not to be confused with a fracture that has an overlying wound, which may not require antibiotics.

Pre-hospital management of fractures is an area that is especially important. Remember pharmacological pain relief does not affect diagnosis (as with abdominal pain where it will be definitively diagnosed with scans and blood test.

References and Further Reading

Greaves, I. and Porter, K. (2007). *Oxford Handbook of Pre-Hospital Care*. Oxford: Oxford University Press.

Gregory, P. and Mursell, I. (2010). *Manual of Clinical Paramedic Procedures*. Chichester: Wiley Blackwell.

Gregory, P. and Ward, A. (2010). *Sanders' Paramedic Textbook*. Edinburgh: Mosby Elsevier.

Hammond, B.B. and Zimmermann, P.G. (2013). *Sheehy's Manual of Emergency Care*, 7e. Missouri: Mosby.

Royal College of Surgeons of Edinburgh (2019). *Generic Core Material: Prehospital Emergency Care Course*. Edinburgh: Royal College of Surgeons of Edinburgh.

Splintage

In the pre-hospital setting, a paramedic may choose to splint a fracture or a dislocation to reduce movement of the limp or joint, which will reduce pain. Splints also play a role in reducing blood loss, chance of fat embolism and soft tissue damage. There are many different options available, but here we will get through a few basics.

Vacuum splint

Vacuum splints are applied for bony injuries to reduce movement. Before and after it is applied, you should reassess the limb for any neurovascular compromise as splinting can cause this.

A benefit of a vacuum splint is there are malleable and so can be applied in the position the patient puts the limb in themselves, as this will usually be the most comfortable. Splinting the limb in position should be considered unless:

- Gross limb deformity unless has been reduced and requires to be kept in position
- Tenting of the skin (bone nearly breaching skin layer
- Loss of distal pulse

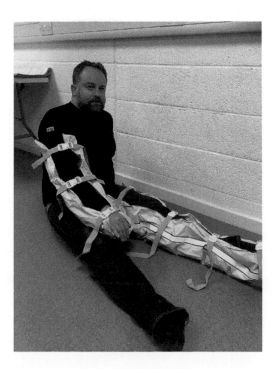

Figure 2.14 Vacuum splints.

Box splint

- Provides rigid security for fractures
- Fixed position requiring patient to fit splint and not splint to patient

Traction splint

A traction splint is typically applied to a mid-shaft femur fracture although some specialist teams and in certain circumstances they can be used elsewhere pre-hospitally. One of the most commonly used traction splint devices in the UK is the Kendrick Traction Splint. Unlike some other traction devices, the Kendrick can be used in patients with pelvic injuries as well as mid-shaft femur fractures. Here, we will discuss how to apply the device.

1. Gain consent from the patient after explaining the procedure (when appropriate)
2. Provide analgesia
3. Ensure the equipment is serviceable, clean and undamaged.
4. Apply manual traction to the limb if there is sufficient help to do so
5. Apply the ankle hitch and tighten the green strap under heel
6. Apply the thigh loop buckle by sliding under knee and working up and tighten
   a. Pole holder should be approximately belt level
   b. In men, beware of genitalia
7. Measure out pole to approximately one section extending beyond the foot
8. Insert top of pole into pole holder
9. Loosely apply lower thigh strap

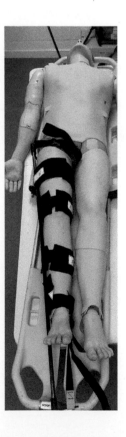

Figure 2.15 Kendrick traction device applied to a manikin.

10. Fit yellow tab over end of pole
11. Apply traction by pulling the red tab to a tension agreed as per local protocols
12. Apply upper thigh strap
13. Adjust lower thigh strap
14. Apply lower leg strap
15. Re-assess including pulses

Pelvic splint

Pelvic splints are designed to minimise blood loss in patients with significant pelvic injury. Application can close the gap between disrupted bone plates but can potentially worsen injury if applied incorrectly or inappropriately. Patients with a high suspicion of pelvic injury through mechanism and pain should be considered. Clinical assessment is difficult and the pelvis should <u>not</u> be sprung at any time

Pelvic splints will not provide benefits for fractures of the iliac crest and may worsen injury. The splint is designed to draw together aspects of the pelvic ring where there can be significant blood loss.

By considering which parts of the anatomy are being pushed together when applying it should help in preventing the misplacement of the device as well as inappropriate placement. The Royal College of Surgeons of Edinburgh provide really useful guidance on how and when pelvic binder should be used.

There are some important points to note as well about the use of pelvic binders:

● When needed they should be applied early
● There is a select group who do not need a binder
● Training should be provided prior to use
● Femur fracture should also have traction if an appropriate device is available

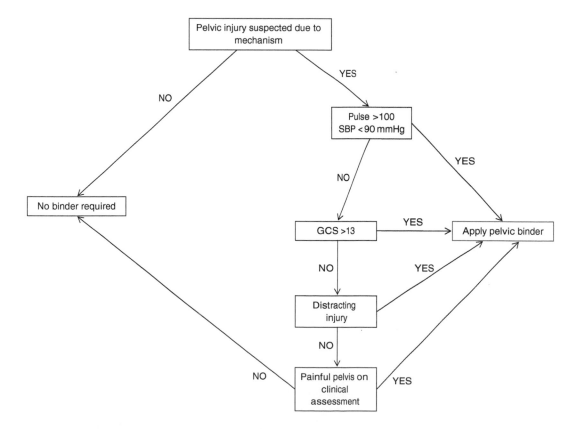

Figure 2.16   Pelvic immobilisation flow chart.

- Patients should <u>not</u> be log rolled if a pelvic injury is suspected
- A scoop stretcher is appropriate for transport
- Pelvic binders should be applied to skin with underwear removed where appropriate

Applying the pelvic splint

1. Gain consent from the patient after explaining the procedure (when appropriate)
2. Provide analgesia
3. Ensure the equipment is serviceable, clean and undamaged.
4. It is a good idea to apply at the same time as applying the scoop stretcher to minimise movements; however, sometimes this isn't possible
5. Line up with landmarks of greater trochanters
6. Tighten in accordance with manufacturers handbook ensuring genitalia is not trapped
7. Bind the feet together with a triangular bandage or similar
8. Note time of application
9. Once applied, the binder should not be removed until after a scan has taken place

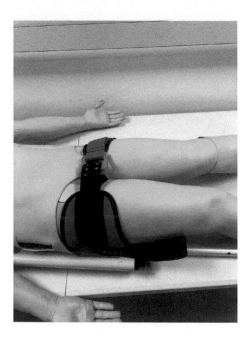

Figure 2.17   Pelvic binder applied to a manikin.

Quick Questions

1. What is a strain?
2. How would you classify an open fracture?
3. How does splinting a fracture or dislocation reduce pain?

References and Further Reading

Bonner, T.J., Eardley, W.G.P., Newell, N. et al. (2011). Accurate placement of a pelvic binder improves reduction of unstable fractures of the pelvic ring. *Journal of Bone and Joint Surgery* **93** (11): 1524–1528.

Greaves, I. and Porter, K. (2007). *Oxford Handbook of Pre-Hospital Care*. Oxford: Oxford University Press.

Gregory, P. and Mursell, I. (2010). *Manual of Clinical Paramedic Procedures*. Chichester: Wiley Blackwell.

Gregory, P. and Ward, A. (2010). *Sanders' Paramedic Textbook*. Edinburgh: Mosby Elsevier.

Hammond, B.B. and Zimmermann, P.G. (2013). *Sheehy's Manual of Emergency Care*, 7e. Missouri: Mosby.

Naseem, H., Nesbitt, P.D., Sprott, D.C., and Clayson, A. (2018). An assessment of pelvic binder placement at a UK major trauma centre. *Royal College of Surgeons England Annals* **100** (2): 101–105.

Prometheus Medical (2018). Instructions for use. https://www.prometheusmedical.co.uk/equipment/prometheus-equipment-splintage-immobilisation/prometheus-traction-splint (accessed 13 January 2021).

Royal College of Surgeons of Edinburgh (2019). *Generic Core Material: Prehospital Emergency Care Course*. Edinburgh: Royal College of Surgeons of Edinburgh.

Scott, I., Porter, K., Laird, C. et al. (2013). The prehospital management of pelvic fractures: initial consensus statement. *Emergency Medical Journal* **30** (12): 1070–1072.

Spinal injury and immobilisation

Damage to the spinal cord whether by penetrating or blunt trauma can cause injury to the neurones of the spine. These injuries can be complete or incomplete and, in severe cases, can lead to death by paralysing the diaphragm and or respiratory muscles.

If you imagine the head as a bowling ball on the top of the neck, it becomes more apparent how the spinal cord can become damaged.

Within the cervical area of the spine, there is the spinal 'bulge' where the spinal cord is thicker. This is more susceptible to injury as at this area the spinal cord fills 95% of the foreman compared to the average 65%. Because the C-spine has the smallest vertebrae and weaker surrounding muscles, it is the most common vertebral fracture as 55% of spinal injuries are within the C-spine.

Thankfully spinal injuries are relatively uncommon in civilian practice within the UK; however, when they do occur, they can cause significant morbidity or mortality. It is important to differentiate between spinal injury and spinal cord injury.

Spinal injury refers to damage to the bony structures with or without cord involvement. This includes 'stable' spinal fractures where the bone segment may be damaged but with no damage to the cord.

Spinal cord injury is an injury that has a direct effect of the spinal cord potentially leading to paralysis or other neurological sequelae.

Spinal cord injury occurs in between 0.5 and 3% of cases involving blunt trauma (such as traffic collisions or sport). Of those cases, 50% occur in the cervical spine, 37% are thoracic and 11% lumbar.

Of the cases involving cervical spine injury, 50% occur at the C6/C7 junction with 33% occurring at C2.

Primary and secondary insults are terms used to classify injury to the spinal cord.

- Primary insult denotes the injury that occurred due to the initial injury causing irreversible damage to the CNS
- Secondary insult refers to the potential injury caused by the patient mobilising the spine on scene with an unstable fracture

To put this in context, of all the cases of blunt trauma, a very small proportion will spinal cord injuries. Of those with spinal cord injuries, a smaller number will have cervical spine injuries (0.25–1.5%). Therefore, considering which patients to immobilise is beneficial as to not put others at undue harm. We will look at selective immobilisation in this section.

Common mechanisms of injury

Hyperflexion

- Chin to chest movement over the normal limits or with increased force

Hyperextension

- Head back movement over the normal limits or with increased force

Lateral bending

- Ear to shoulder movement over the normal limits or with increased force

Axial loading

- Increased pressure or impact to the top of the spine causing compression

Selective immobilisation

Often referred to as 'clearing the c-spine' which is technically inaccurate, the main aim is to identify those patients who are at most need of cervical spine immobilisation.

There are risks associated with immobilisation including, but not limited to, patient discomfort, false sense of security and pressure injuries.

Canadian C-Spine Rules

> Penetrating trauma **without** neurological deficit does not require immobilisation

- Is there any high-risk factor present?
  - Age greater than 65, paraesthesia, significant mechanism?
    - If NO then continue to next question
- Is there any low-risk factor that allows safe assessment of range of motion?
  - Simple rear-end collision, sitting position in the ED, ambulatory at any time, delayed onset of pain, absence of spinal tenderness
    - If YES then continue to next question
- Can the patient actively rotate their neck through 45°?
    - IF YES then chance of significant spinal cord injury is low and immobilisation may not be required

NEXUS C-Spine Rules

> Just because the patient does not require c-spine immobilisation, this does not mean they are free to walk away. The whole spine should be assessed as to not miss the other 50% of spinal cord injuries.

- No midline tenderness
- No focal neurological deficit
- Normal alertness
- No intoxication
- No painful distracting injury
- If they meet all criteria then chance of significant spinal cord injury is low and immobilisation may not be required

Rigid collars

Rigid collars are decreasing in their popularity for immobilising the c-spine for a number of reasons including:

- Decreased venous drainage from the head
  - Pertinent for those with head injuries
- Pressure injuries
- Discomfort
- Difficulty in managing the airway
- False sense of security
  - Collars do little to limit movement but provide crews with reassurance
  - However, they do provide a visual prompt of injury to heighten awareness

Special circumstances

There are times that strapping a patient to a flat and rigid board is not suitable, but you are still aiming to protect their C-Spine such as those with substantial facial injuries. These situations are difficult to manage but can sometimes be managed by providing Manual Inline Stabilisation (MILS) in an up-right position allowing the drainage of blood and saliva into a bowl in front of the patient.

Scoop stretcher

When required, a patient should be immobilised onto a scoop stretcher. This allows for easy transfer at the end of the journey to hospital and can be applied with minimal patient movement.

Rigid extrication boards

As the name suggests, are to be used for extrication only, and only where there is no other method of extrication including self-extrication. If used the patient should then be 'scooped' off onto a scoop stretcher.

Self-extrication

The destruction of vehicles to enable extrication on a rigid board poses risks to the patient, medical staff and rescue teams. Where possible, the patient should be encouraged to step-out of the vehicle protecting their own neck and then lay onto scoop stretcher on the ambulance trolley.

There is good evidence to show that by allowing the patient to protect their own neck there is less movement than pulling the patient out manually. Clearly, there will be times where this is not possible i.e. multiple bony injuries or inability to walk. The fire and rescue service are quickly and safely able to open access for the patient to step out with minimal disruption.

This should only be done if the patient does not have any distracting injuries and no overt signs of alcohol or drug impairment.

Standing takedown

This practice is no longer advocated.

Distracting injury

Distracting injury is such that the patient **cannot focus on anything else** except a single site of injury. This does not include where the patient has another injury but is able to isolate the palpation of their neck.

References and Further Reading

Connor, D., Porter, K., Bloch, M., and Greaves, I. (2013). Pre-hospital spinal immobilisation: an initial consensus statement. *Emergency Medical Journal* **30** (12): 1067–1069.

Greaves, I. and Porter, K. (2007). *Oxford Handbook of Pre-Hospital Care*. Oxford: Oxford University Press.

Gregory, P. and Mursell, I. (2010). *Manual of Clinical Paramedic Procedures*. Chichester: Wiley Blackwell.

Gregory, P. and Ward, A. (2010). *Sanders' Paramedic Textbook*. Edinburgh: Mosby Elsevier.

Moss, R., Porter, K., and Greaves, I. (2013). Minimal patient handling: a faculty of pre-hospital care consensus statement. *Emergency Medical Journal* **30** (12): 1065–1066.

Royal College of Surgeons of Edinburgh (2019). *Generic Core Material: Prehospital Emergency Care Course*. Edinburgh: Royal College of Surgeons of Edinburgh.

Head injuries

It is worth looking at the anatomy of the brain and skull when considering possible injuries.

Head injuries come in many forms in pre-hospital care ranging from a minor skin wounds to life altering, or even fatal, brain injuries. Differentiating these two can be difficult in certain patient groups. We will cover this in more detail in a later section, but it is worth getting the basics done now.

There are a few rules to consider with head injuries:

1. The skull is a fixed box
   a. The skull cannot expand to allow for injury
2. The sum of the volumes of the brain, cerebral spinal fluid (CSF) and blood is constant
   a. If one increases then the other two must decrease to allow for this
   b. This is known as the Monro–Kellie doctrine
3. The only outlet for the brain is through the foramen magnum
   a. Sometimes referred to as 'coning'
   b. Sign of a severe brain injury

Brain injuries can be described as Primary Brain Injuries or Secondary Brain Injuries.

Primary brain injury is the injury sustained at the time of insult, this might be as a result of trauma or medical causes such as cardiovascular disease including stroke. Once the injury has occurred nothing can be done about primary brain injury. The best treatment for primary brain injury is prevention. This is achieved through primary prevention work including regular health checks and strategies aiming to reduce traumatic injuries. Injury prevention is often overlooked in pre-hospital care but plays a big role in the work that could be undertaken by pre-hospital clinicians.

Secondary brain injury is the injury that occurs to the brain as a result of the physiological sequelae of brain injury. A helpful reminder is to think of 4 H's (different to cardiac arrest).

- Hypoxia
  - Reduced conscious level may result in ineffective breathing causing hypoxaemia
  - Reduced blood flow to the brain reduces the amount of oxygen available to the brain tissues.

- Hypo-perfusion
    - If there is raised intracranial pressure then the blood flow to the brain can become reduced and therefore the brain tissue is not perfused
- Hydrops (Oedema)
    - As the brain becomes hypoxic or compressed by bleeding within the skull the cells of the brain can die and rupture
    - This releases chemicals that cause the brain to swell which further reduces space for CSF and intravascular (useful) blood
- Hypoglycaemia
    - The brain is very glucose hungry
    - Reduced perfusion and increased metabolic rate can lead to hypoglycaemia

Morphology of head injuries can be considered as:

- Scalp injury
- Skull fracture
- Brain injury

Scalp injury

- Injury to the soft tissues overlaying the skull
- Can indicate deeper or serious injuries requiring further assessment or management
- Can be minor requiring wound closure and self-care
    - Differentiating between the two is the trick to pre-hospital care
- Vessels in the scalp have a limited capacity for vasoconstriction and so bleed profusely when damaged
- Provide a route for infection
- Easily avulsed
    - Areolar tissue loosely attached to skull
    - Shearing forces may tear a flap of scalp free
- The cause of the injury may contaminate the wound
    - i.e. dirt or foreign objects
- Consider:
    - Was the injury accidental?
    - Is there suspicion that there may be bone injury?
    - Wound closure required and how can this be safely performed?
    - What is the patient's neurological state including a GCS score?

Skull fractures

Vault

- Linear non-displaced fracture of skull bone
- Account for approximately 80% of skull fractures
- Temporal is the thinnest and most commonly fractured

Depressed fracture

- Inward displacement of the skull surface
- Increased likelihood of intracranial damage
- Meninges can become disrupted which increases the infection risk

Basal

- Fracture to the base of the skull
- Raccoon eyes (bilateral periorbital ecchymosis) may or may not be present
- Battles sign (bilateral retroauricular ecchymosis) may or may not be present
  - This is a late sign so may not be present
- CSF leakage from nose or ears

Other aspects of brain injury include:

Coup and contrecoup

Coup is the injury at the point of impact; however, when force is applied, the brain can shift within the cranium an impact on the other side. This second impact is known as contrecoup. This is important as it may explain the neurology you find on assessment. Each part of the brain has different tasks so whilst the injury may be to the front of the head, they may present with neurological sequelae of a posterior brain injury.

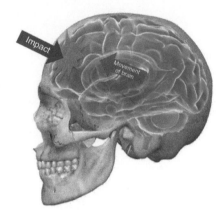 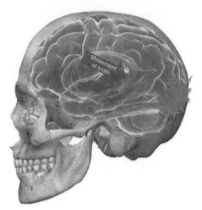

Coup injury
(Skull impacts with
the brain in the area
of impact)

Contra-coup injury
(Brain shifts within the skull
due to transfer of injury
impacting with skull on
opposing side)

Figure 2.18 Representation of Coup and Contra-coup injury.

Focal injuries

Cerebral contusion

- Bruising of the brain
- Caused by blunt trauma to local brain tissue
- Capillary bleeding into the substances of the brain
- Signs and symptoms related to the site of injury

Intracranial haemorrhage

- Extra-dural
  - Bleeding between the dura mater and the skull
  - Bleeding from a high-pressure system
- Subdural
  - Collection of blood between the inner layer of the dura but external to the brain
  - Dissection of the arachnoid mater from the dura mater
- Subarachnoid
  - Bleeding within the sub-arachnoid space that may extend into other areas of the brain

Diffuse

Mild diffuse axonal injury (concussion)

- A common outcome of blunt head trauma
- Nerve dysfunction without anatomical damage
- Transient episode of neuronal dysfunction
  - Confusion
  - Disorientatlon
  - Event amnesia
- Rapid return to neurological normality
- Remember this can be associated with other complications

Moderate diffuse axonal injury

- Shearing, stretching or tearing forces on axons
- Minute brain tissue contusion
- May cause unconsciousness
- Commonly associated with basilar skull fracture
- Most patients survive but may have permanent neurological deficit

Severe diffuse axonal injury

- Significant mechanical disruption to many axons in both cerebral hemispheres
- Extends to the brainstem
- High rate of mortality
- Those that do survive may have permanent neurological impairment

Immobilisation

- Remember the points covered in the immobilisation section
- Collars and lying flat may increase intracranial pressure worsening secondary brain injury
- Those with significant brain injury may also have concurrent spinal injury.

CSF can be difficult to identify when mixed with blood from. Take the time to locate the source of the bleeding as blood can drip from scalp wounds into the ear making it appear as a basal skull fracture. There are blood vessels within the ear that can become disrupted especially if there is injury to the jaw or temporo-mandibular joint, which may cause blood to seep from the ear as well.

Some suggest a 'halo test' or checking a blood sugar but these have limited benefit with easy access to definitive scans at a hospital.

The main thing is if you are concerned there may be a brain injury or skull fracture the patient needs to manage appropriately. Critical care teams carry the ability to safely and quickly manage the secondary insults and can provide this service quickly.

The earlier you call for help from the critical care team, the sooner they will be there and the sooner the patient can receive a Pre-Hospital Emergency Anaesthetic (PHEA) to prevent secondary brain injury.

Quick Questions

1. What is a primary spinal insult?
2. What is a vault fracture?
3. What are battles signs indicative of?

References and Further Reading

Greaves, I. and Porter, K. (2007). *Oxford Handbook of Pre-Hospital Care*. Oxford: Oxford University Press.

Gregory, P. and Ward, A. (2010). *Sanders' Paramedic Textbook*. Edinburgh: Mosby Elsevier.

Hammond, B.B. and Zimmermann, P.G. (2013). *Sheehy's Manual of Emergency Care*, 7e. Missouri: Mosby.

MacLean, C. (2020). *Monro-Kellie* doctrine. Life in the fast lane. https://litfl.com/monro-kellie-doctrine/ (accessed 29 May 2020).

Royal College of Surgeons of Edinburgh (2019). *Generic Core Material: Prehospital Emergency Care Course*. Edinburgh: Royal College of Surgeons of Edinburgh.

Patient assessment

Patient assessment can be a tricky thing to master but will make up most of the job you do. This is by no means a definitive list of how to assess every patient but should give you a framework to build upon during practice. If you ever get lost during a patient assessment, it should provide a useful tool to look where to go.

The patient history is the biggest part of any assessment, as your clinical questioning will lead you to provisional diagnoses, which will then be confirmed or refuted, on clinical examination. Taking an in-depth but concise history is a skill that will take time to develop so don't worry if you can't get it straight away.

When assessing a patient, the immediate aim to ascertain if the patient has a life-threatening Airway, Breathing or Circulation problem. This is called the Primary Survey.

Primary survey

- DR ABCDE approach
- Any life-threatening issues should be addressed during the survey
  - For example, if the patient is snoring due to an obstructed airway this should be managed (see back to the simple manoeuvres page) to enable you to assess the rest of the system
- If the patient has an immediately life-threatening problem on primary survey which cannot be easily rectified, it is useful to call the critical care team at this point to get them moving towards you at night.
- Early recognition and activation of the critical care team will help to bring the care to the patient rather than an extended transfer or admission to a hospital that might be closest but not appropriate
- Primary survey is a very rapid assessment that shouldn't requires any additional equipment other than a clock to count the heart rate and respiratory rate

D – Are you safe?

R – Are they responding?

<c> – Is there a catastrophic bleed that needs immediate attention?

A – Is it clear, can you hear any noises?

B – Are they breathing, Rate <10 or >30

C – Have they got a pulse, is it peripheral or carotid only, HR <50 or >100

D – Are they talking coherently?

E – Are there any obvious injuries requiring immediate assistance?

The whole survey should take approx. 45–60 seconds

Secondary survey

If the primary survey does not identify any immediately life-threating pathology, then you can progress to a secondary survey. For trauma, this is done immediately after the primary survey however for medical conditions. It is normally done after the history has been taken and clinical questioning has been done. A more in-depth look at assessment is covered later in the book and trauma assessment will covered in this section. The secondary survey will also include taking observations

Questioning

With experience, your questioning will focus more around the clinical condition that will be gleaned from the history-taking; however, when staring in clinical practice, it is useful to have a framework to help you remember some of the points to look for.

The medical model for assessment follows a pattern that will become familiar with use and will help to build your assessment before getting 'hands on'.

Presenting Complaint (PC)

- What is the reason for the patient seeking help?

History of Presenting Complaint (HxPC)

- This is where you find out the background to them seeking help
- When did it start, what were they doing, what has lead them to the position they are in
- What have they done for self-care

Allergies

- Is the patient allergic to anything?
- Medications, food or otherwise
- Do not use abbreviations for allergies as this is pertinent information

Past Medical History (PMHx)

- Do they have any medical problems?
- Be aware this information may not be forthcoming as patients may not feel they 'suffer' with anything because they are medicated for it or have had it operated on
- This should include any previous surgeries

Drug History (DHx)

- Does the patient take any regular medication prescribed by their GP and dosages?
- Is the patient taking any medication over the counter?
  - These can interfere with prescribed medications and their GP may not be aware they are taking them
  - This includes supplements

Social History (SHx)

- What social support does the patient have
- Who do they live with?
- What is their mobility like?
- What is their home like?
- Are there any hazards at home
- Can they manage the stairs?
- Are they able to undertake all their own tasks of daily living i.e. shopping, cooking, cleaning etc.?

> Social history is really important as the hospital staff will not have seen the patients' home but you will. Being able to provide a picture as to the patients' function will provide real tangible benefits to the receiving hospital. It will also allow crews who subsequently attend a patient to monitor for any improvement or decline in the patients' status

You can then move onto more guided questions regarding their presenting complaint. It is helpful to document in a similar format to the medical model, as this is how the patient will be 'clerked' by the medical teams on admission so having all the information to hand is very useful.

Observations can be taken simultaneously with questioning; however, it is important to make sure you listen to the answers being given and do not get distracted by the observations. With time and experience, the history will lead you to suspect a problem that will then be confirmed with the observations rather than the other way around.

Pain

Two useful acronyms to remember focused questioning regarding pain are PQRST or OLDCARTS

P – Provocation
- What, where you doing? When it started/it happened?

Q – Quality
- What does the pain feel like?

R – Relief and Radiation
- Does it go anywhere else?

- Does anything make it better or any worse?

S – Severity
- Rate the pain on a score on 1–10

T – Time
- How long has the pain lasted?

- Rapid onset or slow build up?

O – Onset
- When did it start?

L – Location
- Where is the pain

D – Duration
- Does it come and go? How long?

C – Characteristics
- What does it feel like? Any radiating pain?

A – Aggravating factors
- Does anything make the pain worse?

R – Relieving factors
- Does anything make the pain better?

T – Treatment
- Patient positioning and pain relief

S – Score
- Mild, Moderate or Severe?

Be aware that pain is subjective which means that each patient will describe their pain to their own scale. Be very wary of judging the pain for yourself as each patient will present differently. Also, remember if there is pain then analgesia is a stepwise approach.

References and Further Reading

Bickley, L.S. (2013). *Bates' Guide to Physical Examination and History Taking*, 11e. Philidelphia: Wolters Kluwer.

Douglas, G., Nicol, F., and Robertson, C. (2013). *Macleod's Clinical Examination*, 13e. Edinburgh: Churchill Livingstone Elsevier.

Greaves, I. and Porter, K. (2007). *Oxford Handbook of Pre-Hospital Care*. Oxford: Oxford University Press.

Gregory, P. and Ward, A. (2010). *Sanders' Paramedic Textbook*. Edinburgh: Mosby Elsevier.

Hammond, B.B. and Zimmermann, P.G. (2013). *Sheehy's Manual of Emergency Care*, 7e. Missouri: Mosby.

Royal College of Surgeons of Edinburgh (2019). *Generic Core Material: Prehospital Emergency Care Course*. Edinburgh: Royal College of Surgeons of Edinburgh.

Rushforth, H. (2009). *Assessment Made Incredibly Easy!* Philidelphia: Wolters Kluwer.

Trauma assessment

Whilst Major trauma is not particularly common in the UK, there are some basic principles to consider early in the management. Not all major trauma will occur due to motor vehicle accidents or high-energy insult. Many patients, especially the elderly, can sustain critical injuries from a simple fall. We will cover trauma in more depth later in the book but here are some basics points to help you get started. We will cover aspects such as traumatic cardiac arrest later in the book.

Primary survey

D<c>R<c>ABC (noticing a pattern yet?)

> As with everything, early recognition and calling for help from the critical care team is key here.

- DR ABCDE approach
- As before any life-threatening issues should be addressed during the survey
- Early recognition and calling for the critical care team is vital in ensuring best care for the patient

D – Are you safe? With trauma this is especially important. Wearing PPE?

R – Are they responding?

<c> – Is there a catastrophic bleed that needs immediate attention?

A – Is it clear, can you hear any noises? Adjunct or manoeuvre needed?

B – Are they breathing, Rate <10 or >30

C – Have they got a pulse, is it peripheral or carotid only, HR <50 or >100

D – Are they talking coherently? Are their eyes open?

E – Are there any obvious injuries requiring immediate assistance?

> The whole survey should take approx. 45–60 seconds

Secondary survey

Airway

- Beware of C-spine damage
- Look for obvious debris
- Palpate mandible (is it stable?)

- Administer high flow oxygen 100% 15L/min
- SpO$_2$ monitoring

Breathing

- Can the patient speak full sentences?
- Rate
- Effort, efficacy and efficiency
- Support as necessary
- Chest examination using a model such as FLAPS or RIPPAS

FLAPS

Feel (chest wall for integrity)

Look (movement, symmetry, wounds)

Auscultate (listen with stethoscope)

Percuss (may not be useful if noisy)

Sides and back (don't forget them)

RIPPAS

Rate (respiratory rate)

Inspect (movement, symmetry, wounds)

Percuss (may not be useful)

Palpate (tenderness and integrity)

Auscultate (listen with stethoscope)

Sides and back (don't forget)

TWELVE

Tracheal deviation (late sign of pneumothorax)

Wounds (visible, open, bleeding)

Emphysema [surgical] (air in subcutaneous tissues)

Laryngeal fracture (stable?)

Veins (distended neck veins?)

Enhanced care needs (call for help if these are found)

Circulation

- External haemorrhage (compressible or non-compressible)
- Appearance (colour, diaphoretic, shock)
- Pulse (rate, rhythm, volume, location, equal bilaterally?)
- Blood pressure (high or low)
- Capillary refill time (>three seconds centrally)

Disability

- AVPU
- Pupil response
- Posture (decorticate/decerebrate?)
- Seizures
- GCS (especially best motor score found)

Exposure

- Assess abdomen for obvious wounds, bruising, guarding or tenderness
- Pelvis, is it painful? Do <u>NOT</u> spring the pelvis

- Lower limbs (obvious deformity, injury or pain)
- Upper limbs (obvious deformity, injury or pain)

If you get lost or stuck then revert back to ABCDE.

Remember to keep reassessing as things can change rapidly.

References and Further Reading

Greaves, I. and Porter, K. (2007). *Oxford Handbook of Pre-Hospital Care*. Oxford: Oxford University Press.
Greaves, I., Porter, K., and Wright, C. (2018). *Trauma Care Pre-Hospital Manual*. London: CRC Press.
Gregory, P. and Ward, A. (2010). *Sanders' Paramedic Textbook*. Edinburgh: Mosby Elsevier.
Hammond, B.B. and Zimmermann, P.G. (2013). *Sheehy's Manual of Emergency Care*, 7e. Missouri: Mosby.
National Institute for Health and Care Excellence (2016). Major trauma: assessment and initial management. National Institute for Health and Care Excellence [online].
Pilbery, R. and Lethbridge, K. (2019). *Ambulance Care Practice*, 2e. Bridgewater: Class Professional Publishing.
Royal College of Surgeons of Edinburgh (2019). *Generic Core Material: Prehospital Emergency Care Course*. Edinburgh: Royal College of Surgeons of Edinburgh.
Willis, S. and Dalrymple, R. (2020). *Fundamentals of Paramedic Practice: A Systems Approach*, 2e. Oxford: Wiley Blackwell.

Glasgow Coma Scale (GCS)

The Glasgow coma scale is used to assess a patient's neurological state. It is broken into three sections with a maximum score of fifteen; there is no score of zero as even a dead body can score three!

Motor

6- Obeys commands
5- Localises pain
4- Withdraws from pain
3- Abnormal flexion (decerebrate)
2- Extensor response (decorticate)
1- No response

Verbal

5- Orientated
4- Confused
3- Inappropriate words
2- Incomprehensible sounds
1- No verbal response

Eyes

4- Spontaneous opening
3- Open to speech
2- Open to pain
1- No eye opening

There are a few points about the GCS that are worth noting

- Eyes open does not mean simply that the eyelids are parted but the eyes should have purposeful movements in the aim of tracking and tracing an object
- Painful stimuli should be performed above the clavicle in trauma in case of spinal injury
- GCS was designed for patients with brain injuries; although it is applied to a wider range of patients it has a more limited sensitivity and specificity for pathologies.

This will be used extensively in practice so it is worthwhile spending some time to learn it but having it written down somewhere never hurts

References and Further Reading

Greaves, I. and Porter, K. (2007). *Oxford Handbook of Pre-Hospital Care*. Oxford: Oxford University Press.

Gregory, P. and Ward, A. (2010). *Sanders' Paramedic Textbook*. Edinburgh: Mosby Elsevier.

Royal College of Surgeons of Edinburgh (2019). *Generic Core Material: Prehospital Emergency Care Course*. Edinburgh: Royal College of Surgeons of Edinburgh.

Teasdale, G. and Jennett, B. (1974). Assessment of coma and impaired consciousness. a practical scale. *Lancet* **13** (2): 81–84.

Contents

In this section, we will look at the basics of drug administration and pharmacology. This will be studied in greater detail, but this should provide a basis for you to start from. Medicines form an integral part of being a pre-hospital clinician there are many non-pharmacological interventions that can be performed to help patients. An example of this would be by splinting a broken limb would reduce the movement and therefore reduce their requirement for painkillers. By reducing the dose, you can potentially reduce the risk of harmful side-effects.

Pharmacology

The basics of pharmacology involve two streams, where the drugs work within our bodies and what our bodies do to them.

The study of what the drug does to the body is described as *pharmacodynamics,* and the study of what the body does to the drug is *pharmacokinetics*. Each has a handy acronym to help remember the basics, RICE and ADME.

We will cover pharmacology in greater detail later, but here are some basics.

Pharmacodynamics

R – Receptors
I – Ion Channels
C – Carriers molecules
E – Enzymes

The Paramedic Revision Guide, First Edition. David W. Thom.
© 2021 John Wiley & Sons Ltd. Published 2021 by John Wiley & Sons Ltd.

When the drug reaches its site, it will then exert its effect. This can either be to activate a response of prevent a response. This is described as the drug being an agonist or an antagonist.

Agonist – Activates a response ('starts')
Antagonist – Prevents a response ('stops')

It is useful to consider these terms when reading your local guidelines for medicines to understand how and where the drugs will be working. Later when discussing drugs in more detail as well as physiology, it will make more sense why some drugs work better than others or they work differently in different situations.

Pharmacokinetics

A – Absorption
D – Distribution
M – Metabolism
E – Excretion

Absorption – First, the drug must be 'moved' into the systemic circulation (unless the drug is designed only to work on the skin). This depends on a number of factors including how the drug is administered and how the drug is made up. This is bypassed if the medication is administered directly into the vein.

Distribution – Once absorbed, the drug must then be transported to the target site ('RICE') to exert its effect. Many factors can have an effect on this section, but we will cover that later.

Metabolism – Once the drug has exerted its effect, the body will seek to break the drug down. Some drugs will be partially metabolised before they can reach the target site, and some drugs require the body to break them down before they can exert their effects. Some drugs are not metabolised at all but are removed by the body unchanged.

Excretion – To remove the drug from the body, it must be excreted. There are many routes of excretion including in the urine and faeces.

Administration

To safely administer medications, there are a few things to consider, and these are referred to as the five rights: right drug, the right dose, the right route and the right time. This will ensure you are treating the patient safely, effectively and appropriately.

Once you have decided that administering a medication is the treatment required, there are a few steps to ensure the safe process.

1. Gain consent from the patient
    a. If the patient is unable to provide consent, then you must act in the patient's best interest
    b. If a patient with capacity refuses consent, then you must not administer the drug
2. Check if the patient has any allergies
    a. Would this preclude the medication you want to use
3. Check you have selected a drug that is indicated
    a. It is useful the 'sense check' with someone that you are treating the right condition
4. Identify any contra-indications or cautions
    a. If there is a contra-indication, then do not administer and seek an alternative or further help
    b. Cautions can include if the patient has already taken some of a drug and might be close to the max daily dose of the medication
    c. Over-the-counter medications may interact with drugs, but the patient may not remember to tell you they are taking them so always ask

5. Explain the risks, benefits and side-effects
   a. This allows the patient to make an informed choice
6. Check you have selected the right drug from the bag
   a. On a busy scene it is easy to pick up the wrong medication
7. Check the medication
   a. Expiry date
   b. Packaging integrity
   c. Dose/strength of the medication
   d. If fluid then check for precipitation, crystals or discolouration
8. Double check
9. Buddy check
   a. Use your crewmate, the patient or a bystander to check the medication
   b. This will reduce errors
   c. It is worth saying the dose you intend to give any why
10. Check you have all the equipment for the intended route of administration

Routes

Topical – Applied to the skin to be absorbed and act locally (i.e. local anaesthetic creams)

Transdermal – Applied to the skin to be absorbed into systemic circulation (i.e. patches)

Eneteral – Absorbed using the alimentary canal (i.e. oral medications)

Paraenteral – Not absorbed by the alimentary canal requiring a breach of the skin (i.e. intravenous, intramuscular, subcutaneous and intraosseous)

Mucosal – Absorbed through a mucosal membrane (i.e. intra-nasal, rectal, buccal and sublingual)

Time taken to reach systemic circulation

- Oral = 30–40 minutes
- Sublingual = two to three minutes
- Buccal = two to three minutes
- Rectal = 5–15 minutes
- Intramuscular = 15–20 minutes
- Subcutaneous = 30–40 minutes
- Nebulisation = two to five minutes
- Intravenous = immediate effect
- Intraosseous = immediate effect

> These rates are a rough guide as are influenced by other factors such as the chemical make up of the medication and the patient's cardiovascular status.

Paramedics, medicines and the law

Patient Group Direction (PGD) – A written direction that allows the supply and/or administration of a specified medicine or medicines, by named authorised health professionals, to a well-defined group of patients requiring treatment of a specific condition. (*Royal Pharmaceutical Society [RPS] 2019, p6*).

Patient Specific Direction (PSD) – An instruction from a doctor, dentist or other independent prescriber for a medicine to be supplied or administered to a named patient after the prescriber has assessed that patient on an individual basis, e.g. written direction in patient's notes. (*RPS 2019, p6*)

Exemption – Specific medicines that certain healthcare professionals can sell, supply and/or administer in the course of their professional practice as specified by the Human Medicines Regulations 2012 (as amended) (*RPS 2019, p6*).

Prescription – A written order made by a doctor, dentist or other independent prescriber to manage the clinical condition of a specific patient.

Verbal order – These are only used in very exceptional circumstances and must be followed immediately by a written prescription. They **cannot** be used for controlled drugs under any circumstances.

Yellow card scheme

The Medicines and Healthcare products Regulatory Agency (MHRA) monitors all medicines in the UK. The Yellow Card Scheme is the UK system for collecting and monitoring information about suspected safety concerns or incidents. It covers all medicines including herbal remedies and homeopathic remedies. Action is taken to protect the public.

Any one is able to file a yellow card report and it is used to collect information on:

- Adverse drug reactions (side-effects)
- Medical device adverse effects
- Defective medicines
- Counterfeit or fake medicines or medical devices
- Safety concerns.

Questions

1. What does ADME stand for?
2. What are the five rights of drug administration?
3. Can you deviate from a PGD?
4. Who can report a medicine or device under the yellow card scheme?

References and Further Reading

Greaves, I. and Porter, K. (2007). *Oxford Handbook of Pre-Hospital Care*. Oxford: Oxford University Press.

Gregory, P. and Ward, A. (2010). *Sanders' Paramedic Textbook*. Edinburgh: Mosby Elsevier.

MHRA (2020). About yellow card. https://yellowcard.mhra.gov.uk/the-yellow-card-scheme/ (accessed 14 June 2020).

Ritter, J.M., Flower, R.J., Henderson, G. et al. (2019). *Rang and Dale's Pharmacology*, 9e. Edinburgh: Elsevier.

RPS (2019). Professional guidance on the administration of medicines in healthcare settings. https://www.rpharms.com/Portals/0/RPS%20document%20library/Open%20access/Professional%20standards/SSHM%20and%20Admin/Admin%20of%20Meds%20prof%20guidance.pdf?ver=2019-01-23-145026-567 (accessed 14 June 2020).

RPS (2020). Practical guide for independent prescribers. https://www.rpharms.com/resources/ultimate-guides-and-hubs/independent-prescribers#about (accessed 14 June 2020).

Medical emergencies – 1

Contents

As a pre-hospital clinician, there are a number of common medical conditions you might encounter, some will be immediately life-threatening and require immediate management. This section will look at a few selected conditions to give you the basics of the condition and their management. More conditions will be covered in a later section of the book.

This section will cover:

- Anaphylaxis
- Asthma
- Chronic Obstructive Pulmonary Disease (COPD)
- Hypoglycaemia
- Myocardial infarction
- Seizures

Anaphylaxis

Presentation

- Severe life-threatening hypersensitivity reaction
- Rapidly evolving airway compromise, breathing problems or cardiovascular collapse
- Usually associated with skin or mucosal changes
- Can be rapid following injections such as stings or more insidious following eating
- Although skin changes can be concerning for patients, they will rarely progress into anaphylaxis
- Anaphylaxis has three criteria
  - Sudden onset and rapid progression of symptoms
  - Life-threatening airway and/or breathing and/or circulatory problems
  - Mucosal and/or skin changes

The Paramedic Revision Guide, First Edition. David W. Thom.
© 2021 John Wiley & Sons Ltd. Published 2021 by John Wiley & Sons Ltd.

Pathophysiology

- Exposure to a causative agent results in the release of chemical mediators
- Mediators cause mast cell degranulation in process known as perturbation
- Massive histamine release
- Airway oedema causing airway and breathing problems
- Loss of vasomotor tone and epithelial leakage cause cardiovascular collapse

Treatment

- Adrenaline
  - Mainstay of the treatment as is the direct antagonist for histamine
- Fluids
- Oxygen
- Antihistamines if indicated
- Steroids if indicated

Specific considerations

- Cardiovascular collapse can occur without skin changes
- Anaphylaxis can occur without being exposed to the agent prior

Asthma

Presentation

- Shortness of breath
- Usually, wheezy
- Features of the classification of the asthma attack

Pathophysiology

- Immunoglobulin E (IgE)-mediated response
- IgE binds to surface of mast cells causing degranulation
- Degranulation releases of cytokines, leukotrienes, histamines and prostaglandins
- These chemicals cause bronchoconstriction and inflammation
- Lumen of the bronchus and smaller airway narrows
- Narrowed airways restrict airflow causing the wheeze
- Increased inflammation causes excessive mucous production further narrowing airways

Classification

- Moderate
  - Peak Expiratory Flow Rate (PEFR) 50–75% predicted or patient's previous best
  - Usually able to speak unimpeded
  - Breathing rate less than 25 breaths per minute
  - Pulse less than 110 beats per minute

- Severe
  - PEFR 33–50% predicted or patient's previous best
  - Unable to talk in full sentences
  - Breathing rate greater than 25 breaths per minute
  - Pulse greater than 110 beats per minute
- Life-threatening asthma
  - PEFR less than 33% predicted or patient's previous best
  - Silent chest
  - Cyanosis
  - Poor or absent breathing effort
  - Oxygen saturations less than 92%
  - Bradycardia
  - Hypotension
  - Exhaustion
  - Coma

> Any sign from the higher category puts the patient in that category

Treatment

- Salbutamol
- Ipratropium bromide
- Oxygen
- Consider intravenous steroids if indicated
- Consider intramuscular adrenaline if indicated
- If life-threatening then be prepared to start CPR
- Consider calling for help early
  - Pre-hospital critical care teams may carry additional drugs and equipment to manage severe or life-threatening asthma such as magnesium, intravenous salbutamol and ketamine.

> Hydrocortisone and prednisolone are not quick-acting. The primary treatment is salbutamol and oxygen.

Specific considerations

- Not all that wheezes is asthma
  - Congestive cardiac failure and COPD are two examples
- The patients generally do not struggle to get air in but struggle to exhale causing the pressure inside the lungs to increase which can cause a pneumothorax
- As the patients struggle to exhale, they risk not being able to clear their carbon dioxide which may cause coma amongst other complications
- Patients with chronic asthma may have anatomical changes in their lungs associated with chronic inflammation

Chronic obstructive pulmonary disease (acute exacerbation)

COPD is an underlying health condition that the patient may have but not be the primary reason for your visit. During an acute exacerbation, you may be called to a patient for treatment.

Presentation

- Shortness of breath or difficulty in breathing
  - Worse than baseline

- New or increased cough
- Sputum changes
  - Increased amount or change in colour
- Fatigue, restlessness or new confusion
- Wheeze or fremitus on auscultation
- Reduced oxygen saturations from baseline
  - Some COPD patients may have persistently low (88–92%) saturations but during the exacerbation these may be lower
- Patient positioning, may be 'tripoding' naturally
- Barrel chest
- Increased respiratory rate and/or work of breathing
- Pursed lip breathing (worse than normal)

Pathophysiology

- Emphysema
  - Elastic fibres in alveoli are broken down or weakened through factors including smoking and industrial fumes
  - Alveoli lose their shape so patient has to increase the amount of residual air in the lungs to prevent them from collapsing this causes the barrel chest
  - Oxygen has a greater diffusion distance and therefore less enters the blood
- Chronic Bronchitis
  - Reoccurring and long-lasting inflammation of the bronchus
  - Greater effort is needed to breathe
- Acute exacerbation
  - Typically caused by infection
  - Can be viral or bacterial
  - Can also be caused by irritants or environmental factors
  - Reaction to infection or irritant causes inflammation
  - Inflammation, bronchospasm and excessive mucous production narrows airways within the lung

Treatment

- Underlying COPD will be managed within primary care, treatment for acute exacerbations can be instigated by pre-hospital clinicians
- The patient may have a personalised care plan
- Salbutamol
  - You can use the patient's own inhalers with a spacer
  - Air-driven nebulisers may be present with the patient
  - Can supplement air-driven nebulisers with low flow nasal oxygen to achieve SpO_2 88–92%

    We will discuss oxygen therapy in more detail later on
  - If no air-driven nebuliser is available then use oxygen driven nebuliser mask
  - If the patient is profoundly hypoxic then use oxygen driven nebuliser
  - Pre-hospital critical care teams may carry non-invasive ventilation equipment for profoundly decompensated patients.
- Ipratropium bromide
  - Nebulised as above
- Positioning, place the patient in the most comfortable position
  - This will normally be sitting upright or in the tripod position

- Observations and monitoring
- Reassurance!
  - Exacerbations can be terrifying for patients
- May require a pre-alert to the hospital depending on the patient's condition
- Steroids if indicated
- Antibiotics if indicated

Specific considerations

- Hypercapnia may cause drowsiness and coma
- Patient's may have long-term oxygen therapy at home it is worth noting their standard background regime
- Bi-level Positive Airway Pressure (BiPAP) may be useful for these patient's it is worth noting what capabilities your local critical care team have available to you
  - Note BiPAP is different to CPAP which we will cover later

Hypoglycaemia

Presentation

- Blood sugar less than 4 mmol/L
  - This threshold may be altered by underlying medical problems i.e. a patient may be hypoglycaemic with a BM > 4 mmol/L if their body tolerates a consistently raised sugar level. Or a different patient may not be hypoglycaemic until <3 mmol/L as in some known diabetics
- Drowsiness or lethargy
- Unconsciousness or coma
  - Fitting may be present
- Sweating
- Agitation and/or combativeness
- Poor coordination or odd behaviour

These signs may or may not be present.

Pathophysiology

- Usually, due to an imbalance of Insulin to the available glucose within the body
- This can be self-administered insulin or endogenous
- Can be secondary to surgery or medications
- Poor nutrition is also a risk factor

Treatment

- Ensure the patient's airway is patent and secure
- Ensure the patient is adequately oxygenated
- Check a blood sugar level
- If the patient is conscious and able to protect their own airway:
  - Oral glucose i.e. gel or tablets
  - Oral carbohydrates
  - Ensure their airway is not com
  - May still require intravenous treatment if limited or no response

- If the patient is **not** conscious:
  - Support and protect the airway
  - Intravenous glucose as per guidelines
  - If IV access not readily available then consider IM glucose

Specific considerations

- If the patient is given short-acting sugars (i.e. glucose gel or IV glucose), these are likely to have a shorter action than the insulin and the patient risks a second hypoglycaemic event
- Once the patient is conscious and able to protect their own airway, they should be encouraged to eat carbohydrate-heavy food i.e. jam on toast.
- Glucagon is only effective if the patient has sufficient stores therefore may not have the desired effect on patients who are chronically malnourished e.g. environmental factors or anorexia nervosa
- Hypoglycaemia can be precipitated by other medical conditions such as infections or neurological events, once the patient has recovered a full examination should be performed
- Repeat blood glucose measurements should be taken during treatment

Myocardial infarction

Presentation

- Pale or grey appearance
- Cold or clammy
- Sweating
- May be short of breath and/or anxious
- Chest pain either radiating or non-radiating
  - Typically, 'dull', 'crushing' or 'tight'
- Sense of impending doom
- Signs or cardiogenic shock may or may not be present
- ECG changes may or may not be present

> Although the typical teaching is into the left arm, the pain may radiate into the right arm, neck, jaw, shoulder or just about anywhere

Pathophysiology

- Blood supply to the cardiac muscle is obstructed or restricted by a clot in one or more of the cardiac vessels
- Clot typically caused by a build-up of plaque on the vessel walls rupturing resulting in a rough surface enabling Red Blood Cell (RBC) adherence
- These RBC's activates clotting factors and chemotaxic agents which attract other cells and platelets increasing the size of the clot
- Increasing clot size decreases the blood flow distal to the insult sight
- The heart has no direct pain-sensing nerves; therefore, the pain is transmitted to surrounding structures
- The pain causes anxiety causing a release of adrenaline increasing the workload on the heart and therefore increasing the oxygen requirement of the cardiac muscle worsening the injury
- As the cardiac muscle becomes ischaemic and dies, then it is unable to contract and the overall function of the heart is reduced

Treatment

- Reassurance
- 12 lead ECG
- Anti-platelet therapy typically with Aspirin and Clopidogrel
  - Some trusts will use variants of this
  - Patient's may have already taken aspirin on instruction of the call handler
- Glyceryl trinitrate (GTN)
  - Sublingual spray
  - Buccal tablets
    - GTN is destroyed by stomach acid so the tablet should not be swallowed
- Analgesia
  - Opiates may be indicated
  - GTN may have analgesic properties in these patients
- Rapid egress from scene and transport to hospital with pre-alert
- Where possible the patient should be transported directly to a Cardiac Catheter Laboratory for Primary Percutaneous Coronary Intervention (PPCI) this should be done without delay
- Some remote services may still indicate the use of thrombolysis, but this is largely redundant due to access to PPCI
- Be prepared to start chest compressions, ideally transport the patient on defibrillator pads

Specific considerations

- Anxiety will worsen pain so it is beneficial to remain calm around the patient
- A 'normal' ECG does **not** exclude a myocardial infarction
- Not all ST elevation is a myocardial infarction, other conditions such as myocarditis or cocaine toxicity can mimic an STEMI
- The role of oxygen remains highly debated
- Reducing the time from onset of pain to the occlusion being treated by PPCI will improve the patient's outcome

Seizures

Presentation

- Generalised uncontrolled spasmodic shaking and/or twitching and/or posturing
- Rhythmic rigidity with uncontrolled cyclical relaxation and rigidity (tonic–clonic)
- May present with nystagmus, incontinence and orofacial injuries (tongue biting)
- Focal seizures may be present i.e. one-sided, facial or single limb
- Definition of status epilepticus is debated but core principles are as follows:
  - Continuous seizure activity lasting for at least five minutes
  - Repeated seizure activity without return to full function between episodes

Pathophysiology

- Abnormal electrical discharges within the brain
- Altered neuron permeability to excitatory ions such as calcium
- Relative lack of or ineffective Gamma-Aminobutyric Acid (GABA)
  - Neuroregulatory chemical
- Hyperpolarisation of the cells resting potential
  - Increases the resting potential towards the action potential
  - Reduced stimulus required to create action potential
- Greatly increased neurological oxygen demand

Treatment

- Ensure the patient's airway is protected
  - If trismus is present then consider an Naso-Pharangeal Airway (NPA)
- 100% Oxygen 15 lpm via a reservoir mask
- Check blood sugar and treat if required
- Be prepared to assist with ventilations
- IV/IO/PR Diazepam
- IV/IO/IN/Buccal Midazolam (as available)
- If seizures persist repeat doses may be suitable
- Prolonged status epilepticus can cause cerebral hypoxia and brain damage, early assistance from a pre-hospital critical care team may be beneficial as some carry second-line agents such as Levetiracetam or Phenytoin as well as the ability to anaesthetise a patient if required.

Specific Considerations

- Remember to check a blood sugar as hypoglycaemia can cause seizures
- Seizures may be subtle
- Seizures are a life-threatening emergency and should be treated as such
- Status epilepticus carries with it a high mortality rate
- Benzodiazepines can cause apnoea so be prepared to assist ventilations
- Benzodiazepines work to treat an active seizure but do not work as a preventative medicine
- Prolonged seizures cause structural changes that may limit the effectiveness of benzodiazepines, early help from a critical care team may be beneficial for some patients

Questions

1. True or false?
   a. Anaphylaxis can cause cardiovascular collapse without skin changes
   b. Asthma is mainly immunoglobulin F-mediated
   c. A wheeze is always associated with asthma
   d. An aggressive and combative patient may be suffering from hypoglycaemia
   e. A normal ECG does not mean the patient is not having an MI
   f. Glucose is never used to treat a seizure
2. What are the three criteria for anaphylaxis?
3. What might you expect to see in life-threatening asthma?
4. Describe what is going on in the brain during a seizure

References and Further Reading

Association of Ambulance Chief Executives (2019). *JRCALC Clinical Guidelines*. Bridgewater: Class Professional Publishing.

Bersten, A.D. and Handy, J.M. (2018). *Oh's Intensive Care Manual*. Edinburgh: Elsevier.

Bourke, S.J. and Burns, G.P. (2015). *Respiratory Medicine: Lecture Notes*, 9e. Chichester: Wiley Blackwell.

British Thoracic Society (2017). BTS guideline for oxygen use in adults in healthcare and emergency settings. *Thorax* **72** (sup. 1): pi1–pi89.

British Thoracic Society (2019). *SIGN 158 British Guideline on the Management of Asthma*. Edinburgh: SIGN.

Fernandez, I.S., Goodkin, H.P., and Scott, R.C. (2018). Pathophysiology of convulsive status epilepticus. *Seizure* **18**: 30159–30166.

Foo, C.Y., Bonsu, K.O., Nallamothu, B.K. et al. (2018). Coronary intervention door-to-balloon time and outcomes in ST-elevation myocardial infarction: a meta-analysis. *Health Care Delivery, Economics and Global Healthcare* **104** (16): 1362–1369.

Greaves, I. and Porter, K. (2007). *Oxford Handbook of Pre-Hospital Care*. Oxford: Oxford University Press.

Gregory, P. and Ward, A. (2010). *Sanders' Paramedic Textbook*. Edinburgh: Mosby Elsevier.

Heusch, G. and Gersh, B.J. (2017). The pathophysiology of acute myocardial infarction and strategies of protection beyond reperfusion: a continual challenge. *European Heart Journal* **38** (11): 774–784.

Lareau, S. (2018). Exacerbation of COPD. American Thoracic Society. https://www.thoracic.org/patients/patient-resources/resources/copd-exacerbation-ecopd.pdf (accessed 22 June 2020).

Norris, T.L. (2018). *Porth's Pathophysiology: Concepts of Altered Health States*, 10e. Philidelphia: Wolters Kluwer.

Qin, S., Wang, X., Wu, H. et al. (2016). Cell-based phenotypic screening of mast cell degranulation unveils kinetic perturbations of agents targeting phosphorylation. *Nature Scientific Reports* **6**: 31320.

Resuscitation Council (UK) (2020). Anaphylaxis. https://www.resus.org.uk/anaphylaxis/ (accessed 14 June 2020).

Resuscitation Council UK (2015). Resuscitation guidelines. https://www.resus.org.uk/resuscitation-guidelines/ (accessed 22 June 2020).

Royal College of Surgeons of Edinburgh (2019). *Generic Core Material: Prehospital Emergency Care Course*. Edinburgh: Royal College of Surgeons of Edinburgh.

Royal Pharmaceutical Society (2020). Hypoglycaemia. British national formulary. https://bnf.nice.org.uk/treatment-summary/hypoglycaemia.html (accessed 22 June 2020).

Thom, D. (2014). Intranasal and buccal midazolam in the pre-hospital management of epileptic tonic-clonic seizures. *Journal of Paramedic Practice* **6** (8): 414–420.

Tortora, G.J. and Derrickson, B.H. (2017). *Tortora's Principles of Anatomy and Physiology*, 15e. Chichester: Wiley.

Waugh, A. and Grant, A. (2018). *Ross and Wilson Anatomy and Physiology*. Edinburgh: Elsevier.

West, J.B. and Luks, A.M. (2015). *West's Respiratory Physiology*, 10e. Alphen aan den Rijn: Wolters Kluwer.

5

Research and evidence-based practice – 1

Contents

Although research may not be the most exciting part of becoming a paramedic for some people, it is hugely important to the profession and to patients. Without research, practice would not evolve and we would not develop new and better treatments for patients. In this section, we will look at the basics of research and interpreting evidence that will not only be useful for practice but also for assignments.

It is important for Paramedics and pre-hospital practitioners to understand the basics of research so that they are able to correctly interpret the evidence used to guide their practice.

Seeking out, interpreting, critiquing and applying new research to practice underpins the phrase of evidence-based practice. By identifying which procedures or interventions have the best-supporting research that can be applied to practice is the basis of evidence-based practice.

Evidence

Evidence can come in many forms and as such is graded in terms of their level of evidence. This is done well by the Oxford Centre for Research and Evidence-Based Medicine that is a nationally and internationally recognised standard for interpreting evidence in context. Level 1 evidence is considered to be the strongest or most robust evidence with level 5 being the weakest.

However, this does not mean that level 5 evidence is not beneficial for practice. In some circumstances, there is no good research yet undertaken to inform practice; therefore, we rely on the most experienced practitioners to guide practice until such time. Level 5 evidence often precipitates further research leading to level 1 evidence.

Also, just because the evidence is a Randomised Controlled Trial does not automatically mean that it is a superior piece of work.

Levels of evidence

A simplified version of the guidance is as followed (Table 5.1):

Table 5.1   Levels of evidence.

Level of evidence	What it is	Why
1a	Systematic review of randomised controlled trials. Data sets used should be homogenous (similar).	A systematic review takes all the available research papers and both published and unpublished data sets (if a meta-analysis) to collate the evidence and identify an overall statistical theme.
1b	Individual high-quality RCT's with narrow confidence intervals	These provide a good evidence base for as they are tested on a range of patients and are usually blinded studies.
2a	Systematic review of cohort studies	As cohort studies are considered 'inferior' to a RCT a systematic review of their evidence is also.
2b	Individual cohort study or low-quality RCT	Cohort studies, as the name suggests, follows a group of patients with similar characteristics, i.e. age, who have been similarly exposed to a factor or intervention and observe their progress to this over time and compare the outcomes between group, i.e. rates of cancers. Often, they will compare groups by cross-section analysis.
3a	Systematic review of case-control studies	As case-control studies are considered 'inferior' to RCT's or cohort studies a systematic review of their evidence is also.
3b	Individual case–control studies	Case–control studies are observational studies whereby a specific outcome in two groups is compared to identify a causative factor. Due to the largely retrospective view, these are considered inferior. Typically, can be thought of as the opposite of a cohort study as you are seeking the causative factor for a cohort rather than the other way around
4	Case–series studies or poor-quality cohort and case–control studies	These track groups of patient's, who have all been exposed to a similar incident or exposure, have received similar treatment or intervention and/or examining medical records to ascertain outcomes. These are largely retrospective i.e. looking back rather than prospective i.e. planned going forwards
5	Expert opinion and consensus without explicit critical appraisal or peer review	These are often based on lab studies, physiology or 'first principles' but in some cases are the only evidence available

Source: Adapted from CEBM (2009).

Grades of recommendation

When using evidence to base your practice upon, it is not as simple as finding a 'good paper' and applying it. Guidelines such as JRCALC and NICE will look at all the evidence and provide recommendations from it.

These recommendations are graded as to their weighting and identify the type of research that has informed them.

As before, in certain circumstances, there simply is not enough level 1 evidence to inform recommendation so those writing guidelines will base it on the best available evidence but will usually make it clear the strength of the evidence base for this.

Recommendation is graded as followed (Table 5.2):

Table 5.2   Grades of recommendation.

Recommendation	Definition
A	Consistent with level 1 evidence
B	Consistent with level 2 or 3 evidence **or** extrapolated from level 1 evidence
C	Consistent with level 4 evidence **or** extrapolated from level 2 or 3 evidence
D	Consistent with level 5 evidence **or** inconsistent studies at any level

Source: Adapted from CEBM (2009).

Quick Questions

1. What is level 1b evidence?
2. What would constitute a level C recommendation?
3. What are grades of recommendation used for?

References and Further Reading

Aveyard, H. and Sharp, P. (2017). *A Beginner's Guide to Evidence Based Practice in Health and Social Care*. Maidenhead: Open University Press.

Centre for Evidence Based Medicine (CEBM) (2009). Oxford centre for evidence-based medicine – levels of evidence. https://www.cebm.net/2009/06/oxford-centre-evidence-based-medicine-levels-evidence-march-2009/ (accessed 25 June 2020).

Goldacre, B. (2008). *Bad Science*. London: Fourth Estate.

Griffiths, P. and Mooney, G.P. (2012). *The Paramedics Guide to Research: An Introduction*. Maidenhead: Open University Press.

Research

Research can often seem daunting and confusing so the next few pages are designed to help make sense of research and how it is carried out.

Within research, there is a lot of terminologies you will come across describing not only how the study was performed but also how the results were interpreted and presented.

Here are some terms to help you get started (Table 5.3):

Table 5.3 Examples of research terminology.

Research term	Explanation	Example
Quantitative	Uses numerical data points to inform statistical analysis.	Researching the rate of drug errors by newly qualified staff to identify how often they occur. This will identify whether there is an issue that requires addressing.
Qualitative	Uses peoples own words and meanings to develop themes that the inform research	Ask newly qualified staff why there are drug errors? This may identify that nerves or stress may be a causative factor. This could then inform new teaching or training to combat this.
Randomized control trial	Participants are randomly assigned to either receive or not receive and intervention and the results for each group are compared to see if there is benefit or harm attributed to either	Patients are randomised to either receive 'Drug-A' or not. Those that are not given the study drug are often given a placebo so that it is not obvious who is getting treated. At the end of the study if the patients who received Drug-A do better than those that don't it *might* be that Drug-A is effective.
Placebo	A specific intervention or material that simulates an actual treatment or medicine to give the impression of receiving the real thing	Water for injection being used instead of Drug-A. Sham-acupuncture as opposed to real acupuncture
Observational	Where the researchers will observe, a group of participants who are exposed to a similar risk, treatment or intervention without actively intervening to detect common themes.	Observing a group of who smoke and a group who don't and observing the rates of cancer between the two groups. Case–control studies and cohort studies are typically observational.
Experimental	Where the researches will apply and intervention or treatment to determine its efficacy or to study its effect on the participants	Studying whether mechanical CPR is beneficial over standard CPR. The researches will apply a mechanical device to a group of patients and compare the outcomes to a group who received standard CPR. Randomised control trials are typically experimental in nature and introduce interventions to study.
Retrospective	Where the researchers will look back over a time period and identify themes or data that relates to the research question	Looking back through a group of patient's notes to identify what treatments they had received for a pre-determined outcome.
Prospective	Where the researchers will set a research question and then actively recruit patients who fit the criteria to be included in their study going forward	Patients who present with sickness may be given either Drug-A or Drug-B. Suitable patients who meet the criteria will be asked if they want to be involved and if they do, they will be given one of the two study drugs. During the study, the patient's will be followed up by the researches to determine their efficacy against a pre-determined research tool.

(Continued)

Table 5.3   (Continued)

Research term	Explanation	Example
Validity	Validity has many different meanings to it within research. To simplify, it looks at whether the results that were achieved because of the study design and/or intervention or can the results be explained by other methods. This is the basis for internal validity, which has many sub-sections. External validity, simplified, ascertains to whether the results can be interpreted outside of the setting in which they were applied.	Validity is hard to exemplify because of so many strands but here is a basic construct. A hospital-based study looks at the introduction of new type of Video-Laryngoscopy (VL) at reducing failed intubation and finds benefit. This could be because of the new equipment; however, other factors may have influenced the results such as a change in guidelines meaning that VL is used more widely or that because they are studying the use of VL more practitioners are using it outside of the study. Familiarity with the new device may also skew the results as people become used to the change in technique. A valid study will show how these factors are mitigated against or addressed. External validity is where the study may be valid within the setting it is tested, i.e. within a hospital, but because it has not been tested pre-hospital the results may not transfer to the setting due to differences in processes, patient cohorts, operator skill, availability of equipment, exposure etc.
Trustworthiness	This is typically used when describing qualitative data to determine whether or not the authors have been transparent about their methods of data interpretation and analysis to ensure that it has been performed in a consistent and replicable manner.	Typically, the reader would identify whether or not the authors have used, and published, previously validated methods for data gathering, collation, interpretation and synthesis. Whilst few tools exist for qualitative thematic analysis, there are common threads within the research streams that should be evident to the reader Full disclosure or data and methods is often required from qualitative data to determine potential weaknesses and so that the researchers do not 'hide' data. Methodology including independent data gathering by more than one person may increase the trustworthiness as there is less chance for subconscious bias to creep in.
Reliability	This looks at the consistency of results and like validity is multifactorial. Simplified it look at whether the results are replicable and if the test was repeated by another person would the results be similar.	If a study is repeated by a different set of researches on a similar cohort and the results are the same or statistically similar then the study can be considered reliable. If the results vary wildly from the original piece of research then it would need to be looked at more closely as one or other of the studies may have flaws that reduce the reliability.
Bias	Bias, like others, is multifactorial but simplified looks at factors within the study that may unintentionally skew the results. This does **not** refer to deliberate attempts to modify the data to reach a certain answer	As mentioned, there are many instances that can introduce bias. This can be through the way the participants are selected or the way the desired effect or outcome is measured can influence the results. The way the data is interpreted may also introduce bias as well as the available data to the public may only be due to researchers publishing the data, they wish to convey in order to reach a desired effect.

Table 5.3 (Continued)

Research term	Explanation	Example
Blinding	This is where one or more person involved in the study is not aware if the treatment of intervention being provided is the one being presented. It can also be where the person analysing the data is not aware of which set of data applies to which intervention group. Blinding increases the reliability and validity of studies but is not always possible for a multitude of reasons.	Single-blinded studies might be where the clinician administering a medicine is aware whether the medicine is real or placebo, or whether the patient is getting Drug-A or Drug B. Double blinding is where neither the clinician nor the participant is aware whether they are receiving the one or the other. Double blinding is typically more reliable, as there is opportunity to introduce bias if the clinician is aware of which treatment the participant is receiving. Blinding the person performing statistical analysis by using randomly assigned numbers and no identifiers decreases the opportunity for bias. An example of where blinding or double blinding might not be possible is where the clinician must use a piece of equipment over another piece of equipment where clearly, they would not be blinded to this fact. However, the patient might be blinded i.e. during surgery.
P value	These are based on the assumption the null-hypothesis is correct and that the difference between the two groups is not simply due to chance	*P* values are typically considered to be statistically significant if they are less than 0.05 At this level, the probability of the results being down to chance alone is very low. *P* values can rarely be interpreted in isolation and are usually accompanied by confidence intervals and cannot infer overall significance on their own.
Confidence interval	Typically, these are expressed as 95% confidence intervals and will show the range of values that would include 95% of participants within (usually) one standard deviation from the actual mean of values.	If on average patients take 10 days to recover from an illness but a study shows that Drug-A has a mean illness duration of 7 days this would seem beneficial. However, if there were a wide group of patients who take just 2 days or 14 days to recover the confidence interval surrounding 7 would be wide to accommodate this. This could show that for some it made the illness shorter but others it made it longer. This would then be compared with the data for those not receiving Drug-A. If the confidence intervals for the intervention group were wide then it would suggest the data set is less well correlated. This might mean there are other factors to consider. Generally, simplified, the wider the confidence interval means there is less correlation between results. This is sometimes considered less statistically significant in conjunction with other statistical markers.

References and Further Reading

Aveyard, H. and Sharp, P. (2017). *A Beginner's Guide to Evidence Based Practice in Health and Social Care*. Maidenhead: Open University Press.

Carley, S. (2014). An introduction to sample size calculations. St. Emlyn's https://www.stemlynsblog.org/introduction-power-calculations-st-emlyns/ (accessed 26 June 2020).

Goldacre, B. (2008). *Bad Science*. London: Fourth Estate.

Goldacre, B. (2013). *Bad Pharma*. London: Fourth Estate.

Griffiths, P. and Mooney, G.P. (2012). *The Paramedics Guide to Research: An introduction*. Maidenhead: Open University Press.

Institute for Work and Health (2020). What researchers mean by…. https://www.iwh.on.ca/what-researchers-mean-by (accessed 26 June 2020).

Mathieu, S. (2017). P-value. The bottom line. https://www.thebottomline.org.uk/blog/ebm/p-value/ (accessed 26 June 2020).

Nowell, L.S., Norris, J.M., White, D.E., and Moules, N.J. (2017). Thematic analysis: striving to meet the trustworthiness criteria. *International Journal of Qualitative Methods* **16**: 1–13.

Developing a research question

> The only bad question is the one that has not been asked yet!

Clinical questions

Clinical questions can arise through practice in work or education and can be formal or informal. They are used to help justify practice and improve understanding. Provide professional development and satisfaction whilst ensuring safe and effective care.

Types of question

Three-part question

- Patient characteristic
- Intervention or defining question
- Relative outcome

Example:

In an adult with decreased level of consciousness is the loss of gag reflex, a good predictor of the need for pre-hospital emergency anaesthesia?

The PICO questions

- Patient, population, problem
  - Patient or patient group
  - Disease of condition
  - Care setting
- Intervention
  - Type of treatment
  - Intervention level e.g. frequency or dose
  - Delivery (who?)
- Comparison
  - Alternative intervention
  - May not be a comparator

- Outcome
  - What is the desired outcome?
  - Improvement in symptoms or cost-effectiveness?

In traumatic pain is ketamine more effective than morphine at providing pain relief?

Research steps

1. Question
2. Information retrieval
3. Interpretation

Answering a question using existing literature

- Search strategy
  - Databases
  - Search terms
- Filter the results
- Review the literature
- Evaluate the strength of the evidence
- Is there a clinical bottom line?

Primary research

Medical testing wedge

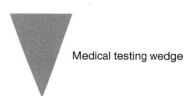

Medical testing wedge

1. Communication and case reports
2. Small scale studies or lab-based assessments
3. Human studies on volunteers
4. Larger scale studies

As you progress through the steps, the number of trials that continue will decrease as some will be disproved at early testing or deemed not feasible for large scale testing.

Costs increase as you progress down the steps.

Questions

1. Define reliability
2. What are the parts to a PICO question
3. What is the second stage in the medical testing wedge?
4. What is quantitative research?

References and Further Reading

Aveyard, H. and Sharp, P. (2017). *A Beginner's Guide to Evidence Based Practice in Health and Social Care*. Maidenhead: Open University Press.

Gregory, P. and Ward, A. (2010). *Sanders' Paramedic Textbook*. Edinburgh: Mosby Elsevier.

Griffiths, P. and Mooney, G.P. (2012). *The Paramedics Guide to Research: An introduction*. Maidenhead: Open University Press.

6

Ethical and legal considerations for paramedics

Contents

This section encompasses some of the underpinning legalities of being a paramedic as well as providing a basis for ethical theory in paramedic practice. Understanding these principles is part of the requirements to become a paramedic and although you may not think about them every day, they will form part of your working practices.

Accountability

Accountability is your obligation to provide a justification and be held responsible for its actions by another party who is deemed reasonably interested.

You are accountable to (not exhaustive):

- Patients
- Family
- Public
- Employer
- Students
- Colleagues

Types of accountability

Professional

- Accountability to your regulatory body

The Paramedic Revision Guide, First Edition. David W. Thom.
© 2021 John Wiley & Sons Ltd. Published 2021 by John Wiley & Sons Ltd.

Legal

- Criminal law: conduct the state considers with disapproval and seeks to eradicate
- Civil law: individuals can exert claims against others
- Common law: laws created by judges
- Statute law: laws created through parliament through legislation

Ethical

- Obligation to act in a certain way and account for your actions
- Encompasses what is right and wrong
- What is good and what is bad?
- What ought and ought not to be done?

Regulation

As a paramedic, you are registered with the Health and Care Professions Council (HCPC) and as such are regulated by them. Other professions may be registered with the same regulatory body or by their own, i.e. Nursing and Midwifery Council.

Regulatory bodies

Regulatory bodies establish standards of:

- Education
- Training
- Conduct
- Performance
- Ethics

As a profession, you will be regulated to protect the public. This is the main, but not only, aim of the regulating bodies.

The HCPC

The HCPC maintains:

- A register of professionals
- A protected title
- Approved courses
- Standards of proficiency

Requirements

- Hours
- Continuing Professional Development (CPD)
- Fitness to practice
  - Health
  - Conduct
  - Performance

It is important to note that neither your regulating body nor your employer have power over each other; however, they can work in conjunction for a mutual outcome.

Professional bodies

Professional bodies such as the College of Paramedics provide a voice for the profession at high strategic levels and provide a platform for enhancing the profession for which they serve. Some will also act as a union for their members, e.g. the Royal College of Nursing.

Professional bodies do not act as regulators but work in conjunction to develop standards and educational policies for their members.

Scope of practice

Your scope of practice is the area of which you have sufficient knowledge, skills and experience to be able to lawfully and safely in a manner that does not contravene your professional standards or put yourself or a member of the public at risk.

Your particular scope of practice is variable depending on the role you are currently undertaking; this may be far beyond what would normally be expected of a member of your profession i.e. Advanced Clinical Practice. Or it could be more restrictive due to a more specialist role without the breadth of exposure or more limited patient contact.

The HCPC details that so long as you are acting within the accepted scope of practice for the rile you are undertaking and you are capable of active safely, effectively and lawfully this is within the realm of the Paramedic role. This ensures that those who are trained to a standard to perform an intervention or role and are employed in a capacity to do so are able to practice legally.

The scope of practice as a paramedic on a 999 ambulance may vary from ambulance trust to ambulance trust around the UK and it is the registrant's responsibility to ensure they are conforming to the scope of practice they are employed within.

Ethics

Ethical theory is part of the role of the paramedic whether consciously or subconsciously. It provides grounding for the actions we may or may not undertake.

Ethical theories

Consequentialism

- End justifies the means
- May have to cause harm to do good
  - E.g. IO placement in a child with Meningococcal septicaemia as this will cause a great degree of pain but ensures early antibiotic administration.

Non-consequentialism

- Unconditional respect for the person
- End does not justify the mean
- Not causing unnecessary harm to a person

Utilitarianism

- Greatest good for the greatest number
  - E.g. leaving an unresponsive patient at the scene of a major incident to assist other patients with a greater chance of a survivable outcome.

Virtue ethics

- What would a virtuous person do in the situation?
- Decisions are made without prejudice

Best interests

- May have to do something perceived as bad for the well-being of a person
- The decision may cause unhappiness but has the desired effect for their health.

Autonomy

- Freedom from unwanted, although possibly helpful, interference
- Capacity to make deliberated decisions and act upon them
- Must be able to make decisions
- Evaluations should be rational

Non-maliﬁcence

- Above all do no harm

Beniﬁcence

- Above all do good

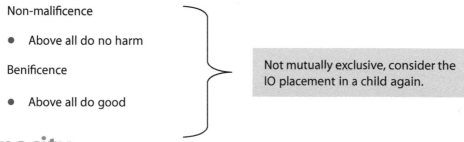

Not mutually exclusive, consider the IO placement in a child again.

Capacity

Capacity

As a paramedic, you will encounter situations where it will be necessary to determine if a patient has mental capacity. This section is a quick guide to help with the basics of mental capacity.

There are a few key points to remember:

1. An individual must be assumed to have capacity until proven otherwise
2. An individual with capacity had the right to make an unwise decision
3. You must take a thoughtful approach in determining if a patient lacks capacity

ID a CURE

This is a really helpful pneumonic to help guide you through a mental capacity assessment.

Impairment – Is there an impairment of the mind, either temporary or permanent, that would prevent you from assessing the persons capacity under the 'CURE' system?

(OR)

Disturbance – Is there a disturbance of the mind, either temporary or permanent, that would prevent you from assessing the persons capacity under the 'CURE' system?

AND (the person being assessed only needs to be unable to meet *one* of the following to lack capacity)

Communicate – Is the person able to communicate their decision to you by any means including verbal or non-verbal?

Understand – Is the person able to understand the information they would need in order to make the decision?

Retain – Is the person able to retain the information long enough to sufficiently make an informed decision?

Employ – Can the patient employ the information that you have provided in order to make an effective decision? Is the information that has been given being used to make the decision that you they are conveying?

Assessing capacity

- All reasonable measures should be undertaken to ensure the patient is able to convey capacity
  - Use of written communication, sign language, translators etc
- A person may have capacity to make one decision but not for another
  - A patient may be able to make an informed decision as to whether they want something to eat but not about their medical condition at that time
- Capacity may fluctuate
  - A patient in your care may begin with capacity and then lose it or vice versa
- If the patient is deemed to lack capacity then any and all interventions including taking the patient to hospital must be the least restrictive option and done in the patient's best interests
- If in any doubt then seek senior advice early

Consent

Consent must always be informed for it to be considered valid.

Informed consent means that you have explained any procedure to your patient including any important risks involved.

Any questions surrounding a procedure should always be answered truthfully and directly

Consent can be implied or explicit

- Implied consent consists of non-verbal but unambiguous response to a question
  - I.e. a patient offering you their arm to take a bloody pressure.
- Explicit consent is a verbal or written consent for a procedure
  - For more invasive procedures such as cannulation or thrombolysis consent must be gained from the patient through an appropriate response.

A patient may refuse or withdraw consent at any time.

Negligence

Negligence is demonstrated where there is a duty of care, breach of duty and harm or damage is caused due to this breach. For negligence to be proven harm or damage must be caused.

Duty of care

- What is the standard required?

Breach of duty

- Has the defendant fallen below the standard required and expected?

Harm

- The 'but for' test
  - Would the claimant suffer the harm they did 'but for' the actions of the defendant?

Quick Questions

1. Who are you accountable to?
2. Why are paramedics and other professions regulated?
3. Define non-malificence
4. Give an example of a situation where you may utilise utilitarianism

References and Further Reading

Blaber, A.Y. (2018). *Blaber's Foundations for Paramedic Practice: A Theoretical Perspective*. Chichester: Blackwell.

Brown, M. (2012). The CURE Test. from: https://mentalhealthcop.wordpress.com/2012/05/09/the-cure-test/ (accessed 26 June 2020).

Eaton, G. (2019). *Law and Ethics for Paramedics*. Bridgewater: Class Professional Publishing.

General Medical Council [GMC] (2008). *Consent: Patients and Doctors Making Decisions Together*. Manchester: GMC.

Gregory, P. and Ward, A. (2010). *Sanders' Paramedic Textbook*. Edinburgh: Mosby Elsevier.

Griffith, R. and Dowie, I. (2019). *Diamond's Legal Aspects of Nursing*, 8e. Harlow: Pearson.

HCPC (2014). *Standards of Proficiency: Paramedics*. London: HCPC.

HCPC (2018). *Standards of Conduct, Performance and Ethics*. London: HCPC.

HM UK Government (2005). *Mental Capacity Act 2005*. The Stationary Office.

HM UK Government (2007). *Mental Health Act 2007*. The Stationary Office.

Willis, S. and Dalrymple, R. (2019). *Fundamentals of Paramedic Practice*, 2e. Chichester: Wiley Blackwell.

7

Paramedic anatomy
and physiology – 2

Contents

In the first section, we looked at the basics of anatomy and physiology and the descriptive terms used when discussing it. This section will look in a bit more detail at physiology and apply it to real-world context to help make it more accessible. Understanding the underlying physiology should help to understand a disease process and how one system can impact on another system to cause a range of symptoms.

Respiratory physiology

The basics of the respiratory system can be considered in two themes, Ventilation and Oxygenation. The terms are often, incorrectly, used interchangeably but actually serve two very different purposes within the body.

Terminology

Ventilation – Removal of Carbon Dioxide from the body (inhaling and exhaling)
Oxygenation – Provision of Oxygen to the tissues

Respiratory paradox

Ventilation ≠ Oxygenation

- Just because air is moving in and out does not mean that there is sufficient oxygen reaching the tissues

Oxygenation ≠ Ventilation

- Just because you are providing oxygen and achieving saturations does not mean the patient is exchanging CO_2

Ventilation

- Negative pressure generated within the thorax to inhale and positive pressure generated to cause exhalation
- Carbon dioxide is returned from the tissues to the lungs via the venous system
- On inspiration, the partial pressure of carbon dioxide in the veins is greater than in the alveoli
- Because of the pressure gradient, the carbon dioxide diffuses through the alveoli where it can then be exhaled
- In addition, the oxygenation of the blood at this point displaces the carbon dioxide in a process referred to as the Haldane Effect
- The amount of air moved in inhalation and exhalation is referred to as the tidal volume (TV)
- Adults can vary their tidal volume according to needs
- Over a minute, the amount of air moved is referred to as the minute volume (MV)
- MV is calculated by multiplying the Tidal Volume by the Respiratory Rate (RR)
  - $TV \times RR = MV$
  - E.g. $500 \, mL \times 12 = 6000 \, mL$
- By increasing the Respiratory Rate or the Tidal Volume, you can effect the minute volume
  - $500 \, mL \times 18 = 9000 \, mL$

    Or
  - $650 \, mL \times 12 = 7800 \, mL$
- This shows that even small changes can have a big impact on the MV
- This is pertinent when using a BVM as by altering the rate or volume of ventilation can achieve a targeted End-tidal Carbon Dioxide ($EtCO_2$)
- Typically by increasing the MV, this will increase the amount of Carbon Dioxide removed from the body
- Usually, ventilation is triggered by chemoreceptors in the medulla oblongata
- Ventilation is a negative feedback loop response

Carbon dioxide generation

- Waste product of cellular respiration
- Cellular respiration creates energy in the form of ATP
- Described in the Krebs cycle

Factors effecting ventilation

- Obstruction
  - Prevents the movement of air within the airways
  - E.g. bronchospasm (asthma)
- Restriction
  - Prevent the expansion of the chest to allow air movement
  - E.g. kyphosis
- Surface area
  - Reduction in space within the lungs for diffusion to occur
  - E.g. atelectasis or scarring
- Disease process
  - Factors arising as a result of a disease process preventing ventilation
  - E.g. sputum or fluid from infection
- Circulatory
  - Anything inhibiting the transportation of carbon dioxide to the lungs
  - E.g. hypotension, hypovolaemia or 'low-flow' states

Carriage of Carbon Dioxide

- A small proportion is carried bound to the haemoglobin in the red blood cells
- The majority is dissolved into the plasma where it can be used to make bicarbonate to act as a buffer
  - This means it can both accept Hydrogen ions (H⁺) which are an acid to make the blood less acidic or disassociate to create H⁺ to increase the acidity

Acid-Base (Bicarbonate)

- $CO_2 + H_2O \leftrightarrows H_2CO_3 \leftrightarrows H^+ + H^+CO_3^-$
- If there is an excess of CO_2 because there is insufficient ventilation (retention) or excessive CO_2 production (metabolism), then the equation shifts to the right and there is more available H⁺ within the blood leading to acidaemia (lowered pH of the blood) through a process referred to a acidosis (production of H⁺)
- To cope with acidaemia, the body will naturally try to increase the minute volume
  - E.g. Kussmuls breathing in Diabetic Ketoacidosis (DKA)
- Patients may be unable to manage their own ventilation causing a rise on CO_2 and a lowering of the blood pH (acidosis)
  - Think head injuries
  - Pertinence of early critical care intervention to mitigate this

Mechanical ventilation

- Ventilation as a result of an external positive pressure
- BVM, non-invasive (BiPAP) or using Ventilator
- Easy to over-ventilate
  - Remember the MV equation, small difference in TV increase the MV greatly
- Higher tidal volumes are associated with barotrauma
  - Consider the size of the BVM and how much you squeeze it
- Prolonged ventilation at high volumes can cause damage to the lungs
  - How long you are ventilating with a BVM
- Use of advanced ventilators can mitigate this with selected settings
  - Commonly carried by critical care teams
- Aim currently is between 6–8 mL/kg of the patients Ideal Body Weight
  - Not actual body weight

Monitoring ventilation

- End-tidal Carbon Dioxide
- Blood gas
- EtCO₂ waveform
  - Vast amounts of information can be gleaned from an EtCO₂ trace
- Ventilator pressures

End-tidal carbon dioxide

Definitions

- Capnography – Concentration of CO_2 displayed as a waveform with numerical indication
- Capnometry – Concentration of CO_2 displayed as a numerical value
- Colournometry – Concentration of CO_2 displayed by a colour changing indicator

Capnography is the gold standard for monitoring EtCO$_2$

Capnography is mandatory if an advanced airway is being used.

Capnography should be used at any time when using mechanical ventilation i.e. BVM with facemask.

Capnography is useful in self-ventilating patients for waveform however the numerical value may be misleading.

Capnograph trace:

- **A)** Start of Inhalation
- **B)** End of Inhalation
- **C)** Start of Exhalation
- **D)** End Exhalation
- **E)** End-tidal reading
- **B-C)** Respiratory baseline
- **D-E)** Expiratory plateau

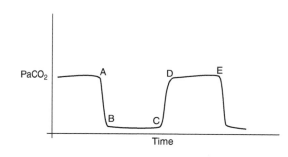

Interpreting the capnograph trace

Normal trace

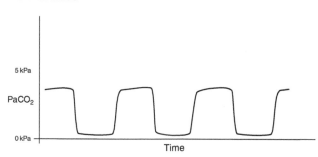

- EtCO$_2$ and RR within normal range
- Box like waveform

HyPOventilation

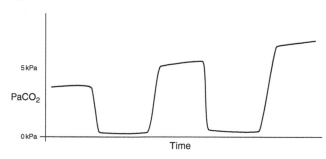

- Increasing EtCO$_2$
- Decreased RR

HyPERventilation

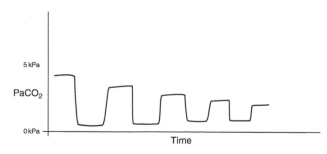

- Decreasing EtCO$_2$
- Increased RR

Bronchospasm

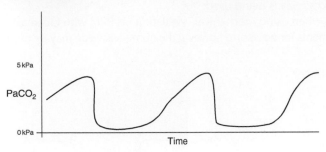

- Airway narrowing
- Difficult exhalation
- 'Shark fin' appearance

Loss of trace

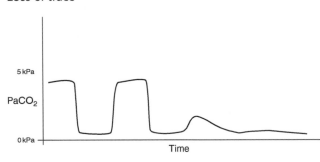

- Cardiac arrest
- Tube displacement

Oxygenation

- Oxygen concentration is described as a percentage
- This percentage can be described using a decimal
- Oxygen as part of the air that is breathed in is described as a Fraction of inspired O_2 (FiO_2)
  - This is typically described using decimals
- Atmospheric air is approximately 21% oxygen
  - Therefore when breathing air the FiO_2 is 0.21 or .21
- Oxygen can be supplemented
- Oxygenation can occur independent of ventilation

Factors effecting oxygenation

- FiO_2
  - By increasing the available oxygen, you increase the partial pressure of oxygen in the lungs; therefore, oxygen will move more readily into the lungs (Fick's first law of diffusion)
- Surface area
  - Positive End Expiratory Pressure
  - Pneumothorax
  - Previous medical problems such as scarring or lobectomy
- Diffusion
  - Increasing pressure gradient will increase oxygenation
  - Increased distance for diffusion to occur
    - Increased distance between the air and the blood vessels
    - i.e. inflamed lung tissue, fluid, sputum, infection
    - Fick's second law of diffusion

- pH
  - Acidosis or Alkalosis
  - Effect the oxygen disassociation curve
  - At higher pH (Alkaline), less oxygen is required to achieve saturation
  - At lower pH (Acid), ore oxygen is required to achieve saturation
- Carboxyhaemaglobin
  - Carbon Monoxide has a greater affinity for haemoglobin than oxygen
  - It is harder for oxygen to bind to the haemoglobin in the presence of carbon monoxide
  - May be present chronically in smokers or industrial workers
  - May be as a result of smoke inhalation
- Increased tissue oxygen requirement
  - Hypermetabolic states
- Perfusion
  - Inability to provide sufficient oxygen to where it is required
  - Results in tissue hypoxia although overall saturations may appear normal

Measuring oxygenation

- Peripheral saturation monitoring (SpO_2)
  - Uses red and infrared light to monitor oxygen levels
  - May not be accurate with decreasing oxygen levels
  - Bright natural light may cause false or inaccurate readings
  - Should be interpreted with the waveform trace concurrently
  - Typically lags behind actual oxygen concentration
  - Affected by peripheral perfusion if patient is cold
  - Can be affected by movement and other issues such as nail varnish
- Blood gas measurements
  - Not typically used by paramedics but may be carried by critical care teams
  - Used widely in the Emergency Department
  - Measures the PaO_2 from a blood sample
  - More accurate than peripheral monitoring
  - **CAN** be interpreted with the patient receiving supplemental oxygen using a P/F ratio
    - No reason to remove oxygen mask from a hypoxic patient
  - Typically 10% lower than the FiO_2 due to dilution within the larger airways before reaching the alveoli

Nitrogen

- Present within the atmosphere and air we breathe
- Inert within the lungs
- Has additional function of 'splinting' the alveoli open to allow surface area for diffusion of oxygen and carbon dioxide

Oxygen therapies

- Nasal cannula
  - FiO_2 dependant on flow rate
  - Usually well tolerated
  - Flow rates above 4 L/min can be painful and cause tissue damage
- Face mask
  - FiO_2 dependant on flow rate and choice of mask
  - Can be drying and/or irritating to upper airways
  - Oxygen can be titrated

- Nebuliser mask
  - Allows concurrent administration of medicines
  - Noisy and can be frightening to some patients especially children
- Reservoir bag
  - Achieves FiO_2 typically between 90–100%
  - Should only be used on high flow's to prevent rebreathing CO_3
  - Cannot be titrated

140 Questions

1. True or false
   a. Normal breathing is due to positive pressure
   b. Nasal cannula can be used at flow rates above 4 L/min
   c. MV is calculated by multiplying the Tidal Volume by the Respiratory Rate
   d. Bronchospasm typically presents as a 'shark fin' appearance on a $EtCO_2$ capnograph
2. What factors may effect oxygenation?

References and Further Reading

Bersten, A.D. and Handy, J.M. (2018). *Oh's Intensive Care Manual*. Edinburgh: Elsevier.

Bourke, S.J. and Burns, G.P. (2015). *Respiratory Medicine: Lecture Notes*, 9e. Chichester: Wiley Blackwell.

British Thoracic Society (2017). BTS guideline for oxygen use in adults in healthcare and emergency settings. *Thorax* **72** (sup. 1): i1–i90.

Greaves, I. and Porter, K. (2007). *Oxford Handbook of Pre-Hospital Care*. Oxford: Oxford University Press.

Gregory, P. and Ward, A. (2010). *Sanders' Paramedic Textbook*. Edinburgh: Mosby Elsevier.

Nickson, C. (2020). ARDSnet ventilation strategy. Life In The Fast Lane. https://litfl.com/ardsnet-ventilation-strategy/ (accessed 28 June 2020).

Nutbeam, T. and Boylan, M. (2013). *ABC of Prehospital Emergency Medicine*. Chichester: Wiley.

Royal College of Surgeons of Edinburgh (2019). *Generic Core Material: Prehospital Emergency Care Course*. Edinburgh: Royal College of Surgeons of Edinburgh.

Simonis, F.D. (2018). Effect of a low vs intermediate tidal volume strategy on ventilator-free days in intensive care unit patients without ARDS: a randomized clinical trial. *JAMA* **320** (18): 1872–1880.

Tortora, G.J. and Derrickson, B.H. (2017). *Tortora's principles of Anatomy and Physiology*, 15e. Chichester: Wiley.

Waugh, A. and Grant, A. (2018). *Ross and Wilson Anatomy and Physiology*. Edinburgh: Elsevier.

West, J.B. and Luks, A.M. (2015). *West's Respiratory Physiology*, 10e. Alphen aan den Rijn: Wolters Kluwer.

> Think about the system as having a pipe going in, a pump, and a pipe coming out. A failure or inefficiency of any one these elements will impact on the others.

Cardiac physiology

The basics of the cardiac physiology can be broke down into three broad themes: Pre-load, Contractility and Afterload; these effect the stroke volume. The heart rate is also a component of the cardiac physiology, and together, all four factors will influence the Cardiac Output. We will cover these in this section and then look at some of the physiological changes that can affect these to put them into the context of your practice and conditions you might encounter.

Pre-load

- Measure of the stretch in the ventricle as the end of diastole
- Directly effects Stroke Volume

- Sometimes referred to as the 'filling' of the heart
- Heart needs blood in the ventricles to pump around the body
- Too much blood causes it to stretch (increased pre-load)
- Too little blood (decreased pre-load) reduces the hearts function to properly eject enough blood around the body
- Can be affected by venous return and atrial contraction
- Ventricles are filled largely passively with the final filling from the atrial 'kick'

Raised pre-load

- Increased in conditions such as heart failure
- 'Over filled' ventricle
  - Does not mean the patient is over filled systemically
  - May be pathological
- Increased pre-load = increased oxygen demand by cardiac muscle
- If prolonged, untreated, increase in pre-load then ventricular remodelling occurs further decrementing the ability of the left ventricle

Decreased pre-load

- Decreased in conditions such as shock (distributive, hypovolaemic etc)
- Decreased blood return to the left ventricle
- Less blood to then pump put and around the body

In practice

- Drugs you can give as a Paramedic can affect pre-load in different ways
- GTN will cause vasodilatation and reduce pre-load
- Furosemide will cause diuresis (remove water from the body) and therefore reduce circulating volume returning to the heart
- Fluid therapy can increase pre-load

Contractility

- Sometimes referred to as inotropy
- Refers to the strength of contraction in the myocardial fibres

Increased contractility

- Sympathetic nervous system innervation
- Calcium mediated activation of actin-myosin increased
- Adrenaline/Noradrenaline (endogenous or administered)
- Drugs
- Hypermetabolic states
- Increased heart rate will typically cause an increase in contractility however after a certain point the tachycardia will impair normal function and become detrimental

Decreased contractility

- Parasympathetic nervous system innervation
- Metabolic

- Electrolyte imbalances such as low calcium
- Drugs
- Myocardial damage including previous MI will reduce the amount of useable cardiac muscle for contraction due to scarring and fibrosis

In practice

- Increased contractility as a result of sympathetic drive seen in a range of conditions
- 'Bounding pulses' seen in early sepsis
- Low calcium states may precipitate reduced contractility
- Patient may take drugs that affect the ability to increase contractility such as Calcium Channel Blockers
- Inability to increase contractility may effect the ability to account for hypotension by other causes

After-load

- Pressure the heart must overcome in order to eject blood
- Proportional to the Mean Arterial Pressure (MAP)
- Affected by factors such as Aortic and Pulmonary pressures as well as Systemic Vascular Resistance (SVR)
- Increased afterload mean increased workload for the heart causing strain if prolonged and may lead to hypertrophy of the ventricles
- Stretch in the vessels is sensed by baroreceptors that feedback to the heart to modulate cardiac output accordingly

Increased afterload

- Increase in systemic vascular resistance such as vasoconstriction
- Narrowing of the outflow tract from the heart such as Stenosis of the valves or vessels
- Decreased Mean Arterial Pressure
- Hypertension (increased pressure in the vessels for the heart to 'push' against to eject blood)
- Pulmonary hypertension
- Aortic regurgitation

Decreased afterload

- Hypotension
- Loss of systemic vascular resistance (vasodilatation, loss of nervous innervation)
- Mitral regurgitation
- At lower afterloads, more blood will be ejected from the heart

In practice

- May observe patients in heart failure secondary to increased afterload physiology
- Cardiomyopathies
- Observing patients with undiagnosed and untreated hypertension in the community and referring to primary care services

Frank-starling

- Increase in pre-load will cause an increase in stroke volume if all other components remain constant

Electrophysiology

- Abnormal electric currents within the heart may result in abnormal cardiac function
- Sympathetic and Parasympathetic control
- Responsible for the Heart Rate portion of cardiac output
- Monitored using the ECG
  - Consider the abnormal ECG in relation to how it may effect the heart i.e. loss of atrial kick in AF may result in reduced pre-load. . .
- Relies on Calcium, Sodium and Potassium
  - Any imbalance in these can have cardiac consequences
  - These consequences may not be overt

Fluid compartment model

- Fluid within the body is largely contained within three spaces or compartments
- This can be referred to as the fluid compartment model
- Each space is numbered for description
  - 1st space – Intra-vascular fluid – Smallest volume of fluid
  - 2nd space – Intra-cellular fluid – Largest volume of fluid
  - 3rd space – Interstitial fluid
- Exact proportions are debated

Fluid shift

- Movement of fluid from one compartment to another
- Largely as a result of hydrostatic, osmotic and oncotic pressure gradients
- If a large volume of fluid moves from the intra-vascular space to the interstitial space there is less circulating volume which can cause a drop in blood pressure

Third spacing

- Term typically used to describe a shift of fluid from the intra-vascular space to the interstitial space
- Semi-permeable membrane of the vasculature
- Results in oedema in the tissues if fluid shift into interstitial space
- Commonly seen in sepsis where the vascular walls become increasingly permeable due to chemical and inflammatory mediators
- Can result from burns
- Fluid shifts can occur into body cavities such as the abdomen (ascites) or the chest (pleural effusions)
- Can result in a form of hypovolaemic shock whereby the patient is intra-vascular deplete (not enough fluid within the blood vessels because the water has leaked into other spaces) which may require fluid therapy
- Shifts can also occur from the cells into the interstitial space which requires more careful management in hospitals

In practice

- Sepsis patient's may be third spacing large volumes of fluid leaving them intra-vascularly deplete and requiring fluid resuscitation
- Burns patients will third space large volumes of fluid requiring fluid resuscitation in line with guidance for burns
- Patients with hyperosmotic physiologies such as DKA may be highly susceptible to fluid resuscitation with detrimental side effects

Blood pressure regulation

Renin-Angiotensin-Aldosterone system

- Renin
  - Renin (enzyme) released from the JuxtaGlomerular Apparatus (JGA)
  - Released caused as a response to
  - Reduced sodium delivery to the distal convoluted tubule
    - Reduced blood flow to the kidneys
    - Sympathetic innervation
    - Activates Angiotensinogen
- Angiotensinogen
  - Released from the liver
- Activated by Renin to form Angiotensin-I
- Angiotensin-I
  - Converted to Angiotensin-II by Angiotensin-Converting Enzyme (ACE)
  - Converted largely in the lungs
  - Some conversion occurs within the kidneys but less so
- Angiotensin-II
  - Vasoconstricts
  - Stimulates Sodium reabsorption
    - Helps to retain water
  - Increased release of Noradrenaline
  - Stimulates thirst
  - Increases release of ADH
  - Stimulates release of Aldosterone
- Aldosterone
  - Hormone released from the adrenal cortex
  - Increased sodium reabsorption
  - Stimulate Potassium excretion by the kidneys

> You might recognise ACE from some medications

Baroreceptors

- Rapid response to rises and falls in blood pressure
- Found largely in the tunica adventitia of the carotids and aortic arch
- Moderate blood pressure by chemical mediators

Anti-Diuretic Hormone (ADH)

- Produced in response to physiological changes within the serum
- Serum with high osmolarity (i.e. dehydrated) will activate ADH release
- Decreased blood pressure detected through low stretch of baroreceptors will activate the release of ADH
- Activated by Angiotensin-II
- Aims to keep fluid within the body

In practice

- Patients may be taking ACE inhibitors which may reduce their ability to increase their blood pressure to combat hypotension i.e. trauma
  - Inhibiting ACE will have the opposite effects noted beyond Angiotensin-!

- Chronic hypertension will alter the bodies normal function to compensate
- ADH will help retain fluid which may present in shocked patients causing reduced urine output
    - Not the only cause of reduced urine output

Heart failure

- Inability for the heart to sufficiently supply blood to the body in line with demand
- Consider the three elements of cardiac physiology; pre-load, contractility and afterload
    - Any alteration to these may impair the hearts ability to function

- Patient's may be genetically pre-disposed to heart failure
- Can be secondary to underlying medical conditions or lifestyle e.g. obesity
- Can be a side effect of medication
- Pathologies that result in the heart muscle receiving less oxygen can result in heart failure through various mechanisms (not exhaustive)
    - Anaemia
        - Reduced oxygen carrying capacity
        - Reduced oxygen delivery to myocardium
    - Hypovolaemia
        - Reduced oxygen carrying capacity
        - Reduced oxygen delivery to myocardium
    - Cardiomyopathy
        - Stretch in the walls can impede on flow through the coronary vessels reducing blood supply to myocardium
    - Coronary artery disease
        - Restriction in blood supply to the myocardium and as a result decreased oxygen delivery
- Pathologies that result in the restriction of normal actions of the heart can cause heart failure (not exhaustive)
    - Increased afterload
        - Increased workload on the ventricles
        - Increased oxygen demand
        - Increased effort required to eject blood from the ventricles
    - Scarring
        - Previous damage to myocardium i.e. from a myocardial infarction
        - Reduced efficacy of the contraction
- Heart failure can effect either the left or right side or both
    - Right sided failure
        - Typically as a result of increased afterload i.e. restriction in flow through the lungs caused by Pulmonary Embolus or raised intra-pulmonary pressures
        - Can result from left sided heart failure due to a 'back-up' within the pulmonary circulation
        - Can result from circulatory overload (increased pre-load) in patients with poor functioning right ventricles
        - Blood 'backs-up' into systemic circulation usually culminating in oedema at dependant points i.e. ankles/legs
        - Not exhaustive
    - Left sided heart failure
        - Inability to pump blood efficiently around the body
        - Forward flow limited therefore reduced oxygen delivery to the tissues
        - Blood 'backs-up' into the pulmonary circulation usually resulting in oedema within the lungs and associated symptoms
    - This will worsen the oxygen diffusion into the blood by increasing the distance the oxygen has to travel from the alveoli into the circulation

- Less circulating oxygen and reduced ability to pump the oxygenated blood around the body
- Reduced oxygen delivery to the tissues will have expected effects

Questions

1. True or false?
   a. Increased pre-load = increased oxygen demand by cardiac muscle
   b. Bounding pulses may be present in sepsis
   c. The Frank-Starling law states that: Increase in pre-load will cause an decrease in stroke volume if all other components remain constant.
2. Describe the three spaces of the fluid compartment model.
3. Explain why an increased afterload might cause a heart to fail.

References and Further Reading

Bersten, A.D. and Handy, J.M. (2018). *Oh's Intensive Care Manual*. Edinburgh: Elsevier.

Gregory, P. and Ward, A. (2010). *Sanders' Paramedic Textbook*. Edinburgh: Mosby Elsevier.

Nickson, C. (2019). Cardiovascular physiology overview. Life In The Fast Lane. https://litfl.com/cardiovascular-physiology-overview/ (accessed 6 July 2020).

O'Keefe, E. and Singh, P. (2019). Physiology, cardiac preload. StatPearls. https://www.ncbi.nlm.nih.gov/books/NBK541109/ (accessed 5 July 2020).

Peate, I. and Nair, M. (2016). *Fundamentals of Anatomy and Physiology: For Nursing and Healthcare Students*, 2e. Chichester: Wiley Blackwell.

Tortora, G.J. and Derrickson, B.H. (2017). *Tortora's Principles of Anatomy and Physiology*, 15e. Chichester: Wiley.

Vincent, J.-L. and Hall, J.B. (2012). *Encyclopaedia of Intensive Care Medicine*. New York: Springer.

Waugh, A. and Grant, A. (2018). *Ross and Wilson Anatomy and Physiology*. Edinburgh: Elsevier.

Neurophysiology

Neurophysiology can appear daunting but just like the other systems if broken down into manageable physiological and anatomical chunks it is easier to process. It covers both the brain and the nervous system. In part one we covered more on the nervous system so this section will focus more on the brain starting with a recap of the basic structures of the brain.

Brain

- Cerebrum, Cerebellum, Ventricles
- Large metabolic demand for glucose and oxygen
- Very sensitive to changes in supply
- Structures largely protected from circulating toxin by the blood brain barrier

Blood brain barrier

- Enables restricted diffusion and some selective transport of vital nutrients, oxygen, glucose and amino acids.
- Protects the brain against pathogens
- Makes drug delivery to the brain problematic

Ventricles

- Cerebrospinal-Fluid (CSF) filled cavities within the brain
- CSF created within the Choroid Plexus

- Circulates CSF within the brain and spinal cord
- CSF vital for protection, chemical homeostasis and nutrient delivery within the brain and nervous system
- Helps to protect the brain from small impacts
- Flow can be restricted or impeded causing a build up of CSF within the brain known as *Hydrocephalus*
- Flow can be impeded by blockages or by compression from injuries such as haemorrhagic strokes

Vascular supply

- Supplied from the internal carotid arteries and the vertebral arteries
- The blood supply joins at a confluence known as the circle of Willis
- Circle of Willis allows for protective collateral circulation if there is an interruption to blood supply below the level of the circle of Willis
- Internal carotids also form the Anterior and Middle Cerebral Arteries

Cerebral Perfusion

- *Cerebral Perfusion Pressure (CPP) = Mean Arterial Pressure (MAP) – Intra-Cranial Pressure (ICP)*

With these facts in mind it is easier to put the conditions you may encounter as a paramedic into context and understand the physiological changes that may be occurring with the patient. This will help you formulate management plans and know when to call for further assistance early.

Seizures

- Homeostatic imbalance demonstrated as a malfunction in the functions including sensory, motor or psychological
- Can be global or focal
- Many variations not just tonic-clonic
- Result from abnormal electrical discharges within the brain
    - Typically secondary to an variation in the cell membrane permeability to charged ions such as sodium and/or calcium
    - Can be as a result of Gamma-Aminobutyric Acid (GABA) deficiency/inefficiency
- Multiple aetiologies of seizures from medical conditions (epilepsy) to toxins and pregnancy (eclampsia)
- If protracted can lead to status epilepticus
- Status epilepticus an approximately 20–29% mortality rate
- 60% increase in cerebral metabolic oxygen demand during seizure
- Protracted seizures (greater than 15–30 minutes) can cause physiological alterations to cerebral structures
    - Internalisation of GABA Receptors
        - Pertinent because Benzodiazepines work on these receptors
    - Expression of NMDA receptors
- May require second line agents or an anaesthetic to terminate seizure if protracted

Cerebral Vascular Event (Stroke)

- Can be ischaemic or haemorrhagic
    - Haemorrhagic strokes can also cause compression of the brain leading to impeded blood supply and secondary ischemia
- Damage caused by injured or ischaemic brain tissue can lead to oedema (swelling) within the brain which can then propagate further damage
- A key aim in ischaemic stroke is to revascularise the injured part of the brain early to minimise long term effects

- Haemorrhagic stroke may require emergency neurosurgical intervention
- Cerebral oedema can have knock on effects within the brain including a rise in Intra-Cranial Pressure (ICP) and cause brain injury

Brain Injury

- Brain injury can be primary or secondary
  - Primary
    - Direct physical injury to the brain from either trauma or medical cause.
    - Occurs at the time of injury
    - Can only be treated by preventing the injury from occurring in the first place
  - Secondary
    - Further cellular damage as a result of the effects of the primary injury
    - Causes can be intra-cranial or systemic
- Intra-cranial
  - Seizure
  - Neurochemical mediation
  - Inflammation
  - Increased metabolic demand and metabolic drive
    - Increased demand for Oxygen and glucose
    - Increased CO_2 production
  - Relative hypoxia (increased oxygen requirement within the brain with the need not being met)
  - Oedema
  - Dysregulation of ions
  - Haematoma or secondary bleed
  - Vasospasm
  - Hydrocephalus
  - Infection
- Systemic
  - Hypoxia
  - Hypoventilation as result of brain injury
  - Hypo/hypercapnia
  - Hypo/hypertension
  - Temperature dysregulation
  - Glycaemic control anomalies and inability to meet cerebral requirements
  - Electrolyte disturbance
    - Occurs after the initial injury and may continue to have effect for days after initial insult
    - Can be treated by critical care interventions to mitigate the effects of secondary injury.
    - Early intervention vital for these patients

The role of the pre-hospital critical care team for these patients is to normalise physiology as best as possible and prevent negative feedback loops worsening injury. The anaesthetic will control oxygenation and ventilation preventing vasodilatation or constriction and aiming to reduce cerebral oedema. Drugs will be carried that can help reduce cerebral oedema and well as terminate seizure activity. If require a critical care team will provide medication to treat hypotension or hypertension as well as infection and other metabolic disturbances. It can also enable direct admission to neurosurgical units reducing the time to intervention for the patient.

Monro-Kellie Doctrine

- Skull is a fixed box which cannot expand to accommodate changes of the internal structures
- The of the volumes of brain, CSF and intra-cerebral blood is constant
- Any increase in one aspect of those will cause a reciprocal decrease in one or both of the others. This can also be affected by the presence of an intra-cranial mass of any aetiology (oedema, haemorrhage, neoplasm etc.)
- A mass or cerebral oedema will displace CSF first and blood second reducing supply to the brain
- If the mass or oedema continues to expand beyond the capacity for the brain to compensate by expelling CSF and blood this may result in herniation of the brain through the foramen magnum resulting in brain stem injury and likely death.
- Highlights the need for early intervention

In practice

- The brain is a complicated organ
- Early intervention to reduce secondary injury is key

Questions

1. True or false?
   a. The brain has a high demand for oxygen and glucose
   b. Cerebral Perfusion Pressure (CPP) = Mean Arterial Pressure (MAP) − Intra-Cranial Pressure (ICP)
   c. Seizures are always tonic-clonic
2. Describe secondary brain injury
3. With regards to secondary brain injury
   a. Describe the systemic causes of secondary brain injury
   b. How might you mitigate these?

References and Further Reading

Bersten, A.D. and Handy, J.M. (2018). *Oh's Intensive Care Manual*. Edinburgh: Elsevier.

Fernandez, I.S., Goodkin, H.P., and Scott, R.C. (2018). Pathophysiology of convulsive status epilepticus. *Seizure* **18**: 30159–30166.

Greaves, I. and Porter, K. (2007). *Oxford Handbook of Pre-Hospital Care*. Oxford: Oxford University Press.

Malek, A.M., Wilsona, D.A., Martz, G.U. et al. (2016). Mortality following status epilepticus in persons with and without epilepsy. *Seizure* **42**: 7–13.

Nickson, C. (2019a). Cerebral perfusion pressure in TBI. LITFL. https://litfl.com/cerebral-perfusion-pressure-in-tbi/ (accessed 21 July 2020).

Nickson, C. (2019b). Traumatic Brain Injury (TBI) overview. LITFL. https://litfl.com/traumatic-brain-injury-tbi-overview/ (accessed 21 July 2020).

Pinto, V.L., Tadi, P., and Adeyinka, A. (2020). Increased intracranial pressure. StatPearls. https://www.ncbi.nlm.nih.gov/books/NBK482119/ (accessed 21 July 2020).

Purves, D., Augustine, G.J., Fitzpatrick, D. et al. (2001). *Neuroscience*, 2e. Sunderland: Sinauer.

Royal College of Surgeons of Edinburgh (2019). *Generic Core Material: Prehospital Emergency Care Course*. Edinburgh: Royal College of Surgeons of Edinburgh.

Thom, D. (2014). Intranasal and buccal midazolam in the pre-hospital management of epileptic tonic-clonic seizures. *Journal of Paramedic Practice* **6** (8): 414–420.

Tortora, G.J. and Derrickson, B.H. (2017). *Tortora's principles of Anatomy and Physiology*, 15e. Chichester: Wiley.

Renal physiology

The kidneys provide a vital service in maintaining homeostasis. Although primary renal complaints are unlikely to be the primary cause of presentation to the ambulance service patients may present with acute or chronic renal complications. The treatment you provide may also impact the renal system so it is worth noting this.

Role of the kidneys

- Removal of toxins and waste products from blood stream
- Water regulation
- Regulation of electrolytes
- Secretion of hormones
- Regulation of blood pressure

Although blood pressure regulation was discussed in cardiac physiology it remains an important factor in renal physiology. By reviewing the functions of the kidneys it is possible to predict possible effects of kidney dysfunction. The functional unit within the kidney is known as the nephron

Action of the nephron

- Blood enters the glomerulus via the afferent arteriole and leaves by the efferent arteriole
- Water, some toxins, electrolytes, glucose, Creatinine and Urea are filtered out into the Bowmans capsule and juxtaglomerular apparatus
  - Should exclude filtration of protein and red blood cells evidence of these suggests disease process within the kidney
- The filtrate then passes into the proximal convoluted tubule
  - Reabsorption of electrolytes, water, and glucose
  - Nearly all the glucose is reabsorbed at this point
  - Uric acid and other acids secreted into the proximal convoluted tubule
    - Organic acids can include antibiotics
- The proximal convoluted tubule leads onto the loop on Henley
  - Concentrates waste products by:
  - Reabsorbing water in the descending limb of the loop
  - Reabsorbing sodium in the ascending limb
    - Reabsorbing sodium will help retain water further due to osmotic gradients
- The loop of Henley leads onto the distal convoluted tubule
  - Further reabsorption of sodium and water
  - Potassium and hydrogen secreted into the distal tubule
- The distal tubule feeds into the collecting duct where multiple nephrons will supply a single collecting duct
  - Reabsorption of some Urea and sodium

> If glucose is present in urine it suggest disease process

Note: Creatinine is neither reabsorbed from nor excreted into the tubules. This is the reason it is used as a marker for the filtration rate of the kidneys.

The kidneys, as with any organ, rely on a continuous supply of blood from the circulation in order to perform their function. Local or systemic changes can affect the function of the kidneys and cause a kidney injury. Changes occur suddenly and rapidly this can lead to an Acute Kidney Injury (AKI); changes that are prolonged or occur slowly over time may lead to Chronic Kidney Disease (CKD).

Acute Kidney Injury can be described in three broad areas, Pre-Renal, Intrinsic and Post-Renal injuries. However, there are instances where the picture may be more mixed.

Pre-Renal

- Hypotension
- Hypo/mal-perfusion
- Raised intra-abdominal pressures
- Acute hypertensive emergencies

A patient in shock may have sustained hypotension as well as mal-perfusion resulting in pre-renal injury

Intrinsic

- Toxins
- Medications
- Rhabdomyolysis (cell break down)
- Nephritic syndromes including acute nephritis
- Tubular necrosis
- Kidney disease

Toxins can be ingested intentionally or unintentionally as well as accidental poisoning

Rhabdomyolysis can occur due to crush from trauma or from 'long lies' as well as other causes

Post-renal

- Obstruction
- Catheters
- Nephrolithiasis (kidney stones)

By obstructing the outflow from the nephrons or the kidneys this can cause a back-up of fluid within the kidneys or *hydronephrosis* and lead to renal damage and failure.

The kidneys play an important role in regulating electrolytes and bicarbonate in the blood. Electrolytes are essential to body homeostasis and normal cell function however alteration in circulating levels can lead to more serious consequences and are rarely benign.

Sodium

- Hypernatraemia
  - Profound thirst
  - Agitation and delirium
  - Indicator of dehydration
  - Can have more sinister causes
  - Rapid correction can cause cerebral oedema and death (manage on ICU)
- Hyponatraemia
  - Seizures
  - Headache and nausea
  - Confusion
  - Can result from ingestion of large volumes of water

NOTE: Renal disease is not the only cause of electrolyte disturbances.

Potassium

- Hyperkalaemia
  - Cardiac dysrhythmia which can cause VF
  - ECG changes
  - Muscle weakness
  - Often asymptomatic
- Hypokalaemia
  - ECG changes
  - Muscle cramps
  - Arrhythmias including Torsades des Pointes
  - Heart failure

Remember: Sodium, Potassium and Calcium are required for cardiac, nervous and muscular innervation.

Calcium

- Hypercalcaemia
  - Delirium
  - Muscle weakness
  - Paresthesia
  - Abdominal pain
  - Coma
- Hypocalcaemia
  - Seizure
  - Delirium
  - Muscle cramps
  - Hypotension
  - Arrhythmias

Magnesium

- Hypermagnesaemia
  - Confusion
  - Bradycardia
  - Coma
- Hypomagnesaemia
  - Tremor
  - Nystagmus
  - Psychosis
  - Seizure
  - Arrhythmia

Phosphate

- Hyperphosphataemia
  - Hypocalcaemia (Calcium binds to phosphate)
  - Symptoms associated with hypocalcaemia
- Hypophosphataemia
  - Usually asymptomatic unless chronic

Questions

1. Give examples of pre-renal causes of renal failure
2. What might you see with hypokalaemia?
3. What is the role of the loop of Henle?

References and Further Reading

Bersten, A.D. and Handy, J.M. (2018). *Oh's Intensive Care Manual*. Edinburgh: Elsevier.

Blakeley, S. (2014). The renal handbook. Academic Department of Critical Care Queen Alexandra Hospital Portsmouth. https://www.portsmouthicu.com/resources/Renal-handbook-2014-final.pdf (accessed 21 July 2020).

Farkas, J. (2016). The Internet book of critical care. EMCrit. https://emcrit.org/ibcc/toc/ (accessed 21 July 2020).

Gregory, P. and Ward, A. (2010). *Sanders' Paramedic Textbook*. Edinburgh: Mosby Elsevier.

Peate, I. and Nair, M. (2016). *Fundamentals of Anatomy and Physiology: For Nursing and Healthcare Students*, 2e. Chichester: Wiley Blackwell.

Tortora, G.J. and Derrickson, B.H. (2017). *Tortora's Principles of Anatomy and Physiology*, 15e. Chichester: Wiley.

Waugh, A. and Grant, A. (2018). *Ross and Wilson Anatomy and Physiology*. Edinburgh: Elsevier.

Pregnancy and maternity

Pregnancy has a profound impact on the body and on baseline physiology of patients that will not only affect their day-to-day activities but also their ability to react to acute illness or injury.

These changes might manifest in the following ways:

Airway

- Underlying obesity
- 'Short' neck
- Oedema
- Increased risk of regurgitation and aspiration
    - Relaxation of gastro-oesophageal sphincter
    - Increased gastric pressure
    - Delayed gastric emptying
- Increased risk of difficult airway

Breathing

- Increased oxygen requirements even at rest
- Breast enlargement resulting in greater effort to achieve ventilation
- Increased tidal volume

Circulation

- Increased circulating volume
- Increased concentration of red blood cells
- May not show signs of hypovolemia until late
- Increased cardiac output
- Increased metabolic demand
- Large proportion of blood flow will be directed to the placenta
- Venous return complicated by positioning as the uterus may impinge on the inferior vena cava
- Potential aortocaval constriction
    - Pertinent for maternal cardiac arrest

Stages of labour

First stage

- Contractions resulting in cervical dilatation
- Contractions will progress becoming more frequent
- May vary in length from minutes to hours
- Membranes may rupture

Second stage

- 'Fully' dilated to 10 cm
- Urge to push
- Feeling of need to evacuate bowels or evacuation of bowels
- Completed delivery of baby

Third stage

- Delivery of the baby to the delivery of the placenta

154

Breech presentation

Breech presentation is where the baby presents with their buttocks or feet first as opposed to their head and is associated with increased mortality and morbidity for both the mother and baby. These patients are high risk.
   Types of breech
   Frank breech

- Hips flexed
- Legs straight up over the abdomen

Complete breech

- Hips and knee's are flexed
- Feet may be tucked behind the buttocks

Footling breech

- One or both feet present through the cervix first
- Feet are below the buttocks

Knee presentation

- Hips may be flexed
- Knee presents through the cervix first

   Paramedics should seek specific training on obstetrics and maternity to include delivery outside of normal childbirth.

Obstetric emergencies

Cord prolapse

- Part of the umbilical cord presents through the cervix before the baby

Shoulder dystocia

- Impaction of the shoulders within the pelvis during delivery

Antepartum haemorrhage

- Bleeding after 24 weeks gestation

Postpartum haemorrhage

- Greater than 500 mL blood loss from the genital tract within 24 hours of delivery

Pre-eclampsia

- Hypertension during pregnancy greater than 20 weeks gestation associated with proteinuria and peripheral oedema

Eclampsia

- Tonic-clonic seizure associated with pregnancy greater than 20 weeks gestation usually in association with signs of pre-eclampsia

Cardiac arrest

- Rare but associated with poor outcome
- Remember to manually displace the gravid uterus to the left to release pressure on inferior vena cava
- Pre-hospital critical care teams may be able to provide resuscitative hysterotomy to deliver the baby in order to save the mothers life

References and Further Reading

BMJ (2020). Breech presentation. BMJ Best Practice. https://bestpractice.bmj.com/topics/en-gb/668 (accessed 29 July 2020).

Gregory, P. and Ward, A. (2010). *Sanders' Paramedic Textbook*. Edinburgh: Mosby Elsevier.

Royal College of Obstetricians and Gynecologists (2016). Postpartum haemorrhage, prevention and management (green-top guideline no. 52). https://www.rcog.org.uk/en/guidelines-research-services/guidelines/gtg52/ (accessed 29 July 2020).

Royal College of Surgeons of Edinburgh (2019). *Generic Core Material: Prehospital Emergency Care Course*. Edinburgh: Royal College of Surgeons of Edinburgh.

Winter, C., Crofts, J., Laxton, C. et al. (2012). *PROMPT Course Manual*, 2e. Cambridge: Cambridge University Press.

Woollard, M., Hinshaw, K., Simpson, H., and Wieteska, S. (2010). *Pre-Hospital Obstetric Emergency Training*. Chichester: Wiley-Blackwell.

8

Practical skills for paramedics – 2

Contents

This section will look to build on the existing skills you already have as well as gain new skills to help patients further. It is important to note that any intervention made should be done with the best intentions and in the best interests of the patient.

Cannulation

Intravenous cannulation is the act of inserting a plastic catheter into a vein using a needle with the intention of administering medicines or fluids.

Indications:

- Administration of intravenous medication
- Administration of intravenous fluid

Cautions

- Shunts/fistulas in same arm
  - May result in arterial administration of medicine
- Lymph removal on same arm
  - Increased infection risk

- Haemophilia or other clotting disorder
  - High risk of bruising and delayed complications
- Cannulation distal to injury site i.e. fracture
  - Unknown disruption to vascular system above cannulation site
  - Medication may not reach systemic circulation
- Right arm if going for pPCI
  - Preferred cannulation site is LEFT arm but if IV access is required an only suitable site is on the right then this should be used
- Frail/elderly
  - Usually more difficult to cannulate due to more mobile veins
- Obesity
  - May be more difficult to identify cannulation site
- Needle phobia
  - Repeated attempts may increase anxiety
  - May cause psychological distress
- Infectious diseases
  - Blood-borne infections
- Illicit drug use
  - May have scarring of the vessels making it more difficult to cannulate
- Scarring
  - Previous injuries or medical conditions may cause overlying scarring

Choice of cannula size should depend on the cannulation site, vessel size but also for the intended use. If the cannula is to be used to administer a small volume medication then a small cannula will usually suffice. The size of the cannula will dictate how fast fluid can be administered through it, however with increasing size comes increasing pain and should be considered carefully to justify using larger cannulas. Furthermore, if intravenous access is really required then any access is better than no access.

To paraphrase an old saying: 'A blue in the arm is better than two grey's in the bin'.

Flow rates through cannula gauges

Table 8.1 Flow rates.

Cannula	With gravity (mL/min)	With pressure (mL/min)
22G (Blue)	35.7	71.4
20G (Pink)	64.4	105.1
18G (Green)	98.1	153.1
16G (Grey)	154.7	334.4
14G (Orange)	236.1	384.2

Methodology:

1. Indication for cannulation
2. Explain procedure and gain consent
3. Apply tourniquet and encourage venous engorgement
4. Check and prepare equipment
   a. Expiry dates
   b. Packaging integrity
5. Select vein
   a. Distal as possible
   b. Large bore
   c. Non-mobile
   d. Non-pulsatile
   e. Not overlying mobile joint if possible
6. Hand hygiene
   a. Wash/alcohol gel hands
   b. Gloves
7. Clean cannulation site
   a. Swab and allow to dry
   b. Do not re-palpate site once swabbed
8. Secure skin and vein distal to site with non-dominant hand
9. Warn patient 'sharp scratch' or words to that effect
10. Hold cannula at 10–30° with the bevel up
11. Insert the cannula to achieve a 'flashback' indicating venous puncture
12. Release tourniquet
13. Advance cannula off the needle looking for secondary flashback in the catheter
14. Using non-dominant hand place finger or thumb proximal to end of catheter to stem blood flow
    a. Make sure not to press onto the plastic catheter itself as this will cause pain and bruising and may damage the vessel itself
15. Remove needle and place within sharps bin
16. Screw the end cap on the cannula and release pressure
17. Check patency by flushing cannula
    a. If in doubt take it out
18. Secure cannula with a dressing with the time and date written on it
19. Remove gloves
20. Document procedure in the patient's notes

Risks associated with cannulation

- Time delay
- Pain
- Infection
- Allergies
- Haematoma
- Thrombus
- Extravasation
- Necrosis
- Thrombophlebitis
- Arterial puncture

> Top tip is to remove cap from end of cannula and place into medicines port before attempting cannulation to avoid throwing it away with the needle.

> Remember the needle extends beyond the length of the plastic catheter so flashback may mean the needle is in the vein but not the catheter.

> Do not attempt cannulation distal to a previous failed attempt or 'blown vein'. This is because if medicine is administered distal to the injury site there is a risk that the medicine will extravasate through the proximal vein injury and into tissues where it can cause serious damage.

External jugular cannulation

- Cannulation of the External Jugular Vein (EJV) is accepted in some services in the UK
- Increased risk of air embolus if performed incorrectly
- The procedure for EJV cannulation should fall within the local policy and training department

References and Further Reading

Greaves, I. and Porter, K. (2007). *Oxford Handbook of Pre-Hospital Care*. Oxford: Oxford University Press.
Gregory, P. and Mursell, I. (2010). *Manual of Clinical Paramedic Procedures*. Chichester: Wiley Blackwell.
Gregory, P. and Ward, A. (2010). *Sanders' Paramedic Textbook*. Edinburgh: Mosby Elsevier.
Nickson, C. (2019). Fluid administration device flow rates. LITFL. https://litfl.com/fluid-administration-device-flow-rates/ (accessed 23 July 2020).
Pilbery, R. and Lethbridge, K. (2019). *Ambulance Care Practice*, 2e. Bridgewater: Class Professional Publishing.

Intra-osseous needle placement

There may be instances where it is not possible to cannulate a vein but the patient is seriously ill or injured and requires medication. In these circumstances, a paramedic may opt to insert an intra-osseous (IO) needle to gain access to the highly vascular bone marrow in order to deliver medication to the systemic circulation.

The most common device used in UK civilian practice is the EZ-IO® device.

Indications

- Administration of drugs following two or more failed attempts at intravenous cannulation whereby without treatment the patient is likely to suffer significant mortality or morbidity risk without intervention.
- Administration of fluids or blood following two or more failed attempts at intravenous cannulation whereby without treatment the patient is likely to suffer significant mortality or morbidity risk without intervention.

Contraindications

- Proximal facture in the target bone
- Previous orthopaedic surgical intervention at or near target site
    - Joint replacements are NOT target sites
- Previous IO needle insertion in target bone within 48 hours
- Infection overlying target site
- Inability to locate landmarks for insertion

Cautions

- Distal fracture in target bone
    - Chose alternative site if possible
- Obesity
    - Needle length and choice of insertion site

Insertion sites

- Insertion sites may vary from by trust and should follow local guidelines, typically for paramedics this would include:
    - Proximal Tibia
        - In adults

- Approximately two fingers width medial to tibial tuberosity
  - In paediatrics
- If unable to identify tibial tuberosity then two fingers width bellow patella and then one fingers width medial along flat aspect of the tibia
- If able to identify tibial tuberosity then one finger width below tibial tuberosity and then medial along the flat aspect of the tibia
  - Ensure you read the product literature and are suitable trained to perform the procedure
- Proximal Humerus
  - With the elbow bent and the arm adducted approximately two-finger width inferior to the coracoid process and the acromion avoiding the nervous and muscular structures of the shoulder
  - Apply local policy guidance and ensure suitably trained to perform the procedure
  - Ensure you read the product literature and are suitable trained to perform the procedure

EZ-IO® needle size

Yellow	45 mm needle
Blue	25 mm needle
Pink	15 mm needle

Technique for EZ-IO® insertion

1. Indication for IO insertion
2. Explain procedure and gain consent if able
3. Check and prepare equipment
   a. Expiry dates
   b. Packaging integrity
   c. Needle size appropriate for patient size and insertion site
   d. Flush EZ® connector with saline
4. Select site
   a. Noting contra-indications and cautions
   b. Correct landmarks identified
5. Hand hygiene and PPE
   a. Wash/alcohol gel hands
   b. Gloves
6. Clean site
   a. Swab and allow to dry
   b. Do not re-palpate site once swabbed
7. Insert needle through skin ensuring black lines visible above skin before starting drill
8. Start drill applying gentle pressure perpendicular to bone
9. Once a 'give' has been felt stop drilling
10. Ensure skin is not compressed under needle hub
11. Remove inner introducer from IO and place in sharps container
12. Secure with correct dressing
13. Apply EZ-IO® identification band to selected limb
14. Attach pre-flushed EZ® connector
15. Flush IO needle
    a. Most painful part of procedure for awake patients
    b. Can be done with local anaesthetic if within local guidelines
    c. If in doubt take it out

16. Write time and date of insertion on dressing
17. Remove gloves
18. Document in patient notes
19. Ensure on handover to hospital the receiving team are aware that an IO needle is in situ

Risks associated with IO placement

- Misplacement of needle
- Damage to surrounding structures
- Infection
- Needle breakage if not using correct connector
- Displacement of needle
- Extravasation
- Necrosis
- Pain
- Fracture

Quick Questions

1. What is the flow rate, by gravity, through a pink (20G) cannula?
2. What size IO needle would you use for a head of humerus insertion?
3. What are the contra-indication for IO needle placement?

References and Further Reading

Arrow (2017). The science and fundamentals of intraosseous vascular access. Teleflex. https://www.teleflex.com/usa/en/clinical-resources/ez-io/documents/EZ-IO_Science_Fundamentals_MC-003266-Rev1-1.pdf (accessed 23 July 2020).

Greaves, I. and Porter, K. (2007). *Oxford Handbook of Pre-Hospital Care*. Oxford: Oxford University Press.

Gregory, P. and Mursell, I. (2010). *Manual of Clinical Paramedic Procedures*. Chichester: Wiley Blackwell.

Gregory, P. and Ward, A. (2010). *Sanders' Paramedic Textbook*. Edinburgh: Mosby Elsevier.

Pilbery, R. and Lethbridge, K. (2019). *Ambulance Care Practice*, 2e. Bridgewater: Class Professional Publishing.

Royal College of Surgeons of Edinburgh (2019). *Generic Core Material: Prehospital Emergency Care Course*. Edinburgh: Royal College of Surgeons of Edinburgh.

Endotracheal intubation

Endotracheal intubation has largely been withdrawn from service except in specialist roles or certain practitioners. This section will cover intubation but more so the goal of laryngoscopy, which remains a core paramedic skill for the removal of a foreign body. Remaining current in the practice of intubation is difficult with regular training, recertification and exposure required to maintain competency is required.

The College of Paramedics recommend a minimum of 60 supervised successful intubations for initial sign off with the skill being maintained with a minimum of 2 supervised intubations for each age group per month as well as an annual competency check. Skill fade is a real concern with regards to intubation and those practitioners who are able to perform the intervention should maintain their competency in line with local and national guidance.

An important part of any procedure is the non-technical aspect that may have the greatest impact on not only the procedure itself but also to the greater team dynamics. Crew Resource Management (CRM), task focussing and tunnel vision are all factors when performing critical interventions. As the task of intubating may require more thought processing than other procedures this may distract the clinician from observing the patient as a whole or other scene safety considerations. Practicing and maintaining the basics of airway management will likely provide the most benefit for the most patients.

Early recognition of patients with actual or potential airway compromise and seeking help from a critical care team or suitable receiving unit is key for patients who subsequently require endotracheal intubation.

Endotracheal intubation should **not** be attempted on patients with a pulse without the use of anaesthetic agents by an appropriately trained and governed critical care team. This is due to the potential physiological consequences from vagal stimulus by laryngoscopy. Please refer to your local guidelines and policies for further information.

Indications

- Cardiac arrest with actual or potential airway compromise which cannot be managed by other methods
- Maternal cardiac arrest
  - Must not delay transport to definitive care or pre-hospital critical care team with surgical capability
  - Must not delay other procedures that may result in the return of spontaneous circulation
- Patients who have received a pre-hospital anaesthetic by a pre-hospital critical care team

Contraindications

- Patients with a pulse without the provision of an anaesthetic by a suitably trained and governed critical care team
- Patients who have undergone a total laryngectomy
  - These patients will have no connection between the upper airways and the trachea and rely solely on the tracheostomy
- Incomplete equipment to perform the procedure
- Where $EtCO_2$ monitoring is not immediately available
- Absence of suitably trained and competent personnel

Cautions

- Known, suspected or potentially difficult airway
- Intubation would significantly delay definitive care and the patient can be suitably and safely managed by other methods
- Intubation would significantly delay key treatments such as CPR or defibrillation and the patient can be suitably and safely managed by other methods

Methodology

1. Indication for endotracheal intubation
2. Check and prepare equipment
    a. Working laryngoscopes
    b. Suitable size blade for procedure
    c. Suitable endotracheal tube, in date, cuff deflated fully and lubricated
    d. Bougie
    e. Syringe
    f. BVM and suitably sized facemask
    g. Securing ability (tube tie, tape or holder)
    h. Back-up airway device i.e. iGel
    i. Capnography working
    j. Working suction
    k. Sufficient oxygen

    l.   Airway assistant
    m. Personal Protective Equipment (PPE) as appropriate
        i.   Mask
        ii. Eye protection
        iii. Gloves

3. Position patient
    a. Ideally kneeling height with 360° access
    b. 'Sniffing the morning air' with pillows
    c. Ramping if required
        i.   Tragus in line with sternum

4. Pre-oxygenate patient
5. Brief the team and airway assistant
6. Hold laryngoscope in left hand
7. Place tip of the blade into the right-hand side of the mouth
8. 'Walk' the blade into the airway identifying structures as you advance (vocalising may help other members of the team with their situational awareness)
    a. Lips
    b. Teeth
    c. Tongue
    d. Hard Palate
    e. Soft Palate
    f. Uvula
    g. Posterior wall
    h. Epiglottis
    i. Suction may be required at any point

> By identifying the landmarks of the airway as you advance you are less likely to advance too far and 'miss' the airway. It will also help when patients have differing anatomy to ensure you are heading for the right place

9. 'Sweep' the blade to the left maintaining visuals with epiglottis
10. Advance the tip of the blade into the vallecular
11. Lift and push the handle away from you in a 'superman' fashion NOT levering on the teeth
12. Positively identify the anatomical structures of the tracheal inlet (may require Extra-Laryngeal Manipulation from your airway assistant if gaining a view is difficult) – again vocalising what you can see may be important for team situational awareness
    a. Epiglottis
    b. Vocal cords
    c. Arytenoids
13. Pass a bougie through the vocal cords
    a. It may be possible to feel a click from the tracheal rings when passing
14. Maintaining direct visualisation, the airway assistant is to pass the tube over the bougie until they are able to hold the distal end of the bougie
    a. Once confirmation is given the assistant has the bougie the intubator may release their hold of the bougie and take hold of the tube
    b. Airway Assistant – 'I have the bougie'
    c. Intubator – 'I have the tube'
15. Under direct visualisation the tube should be passed over the bougie through the tracheal inlet until the cuff has passed beneath the cords
    a. Some endotracheal tubes will have safety markings to ensure when the cuff is inflated it does not damage the airways
16. Maintaining visualisation, the cuff should be inflated by the assistant
17. Maintaining visualisation capnography and BVM attached by airway assistant

18. Maintaining visualisation breaths should be provided by the BVM whilst the intubator assesses for signs of correct placement
    a. Tube misting
    b. Chest rising and falling
    c. Confirmed Capnography trace
19. Holding the endotracheal tube, the laryngoscope should be removed and the intubator should reassess for correct placement
    a. Checks as before
    b. Auscultation of the chest and stomach
20. Secure the tube
21. Reassess after securing the tube
22. Once able document in the patient's notes

> Ensure regular reassessment of the tube to ensure correct placement.

Risks associated with endotracheal intubation (not exhaustive)

- Dental/orofacial/airway damage
- Misplacement/Unrecognised oesophageal intubation/failed intubation
- Tracheal stenosis
- Oedema/Tissue necrosis
- Delays in CPR or defibrillation

Failed intubation

- Failed intubation guidelines are produced by the Difficult Airway Society (DAS)
- Focus on maintaining oxygenation this may be by reverting to simple measures
- Remember to call for help
- Repeated intubation attempts increase the risk of airway oedema and damage making subsequent attempts for difficult
    - Recommended no more than three attempts by the first operator before one attempt by second operator
    - Between each attempt ensure something is changed to improve the chances of a successful intubation on the next attempt
- Use of 'rescue' airways including iGel's to ensure oxygenation or reverting to facemask ventilation with two person technique
- Please refer to the (DAS) guidelines or local policies

Grading of view on direct laryngoscopy

- View is graded using Cormack-Lehane classification
- Standard classification used by pre-hospital and in-hospital clinicians

1) Full view of epiglottis, glottis and tracheal opening
2a) Partial view of glottis and tracheal opening, loss of the top third of vocal cords
2b) Able to visualize the posterior most part of glottis or arytenoid cartilage only
3) Only able to visualize the epiglottis, no view of tracheal inlet
4) No view of the airway structures

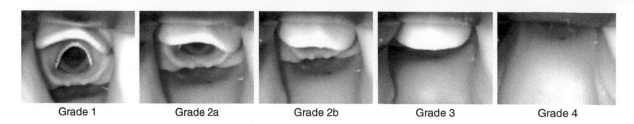

Grade 1 Grade 2a Grade 2b Grade 3 Grade 4

Figure 8.1 Grades of laryngoscopy.

165

References and Further Reading

Benger, J.R., Kirby, K., Black, S. et al. (2018). Effect of a strategy of a supraglottic airway device vs tracheal intubation during out-of-hospital cardiac arrest on functional outcome: the AIRWAYS-2 randomized clinical trial. *JAMA* **320** (8): 779–791.

College of Paramedics (2018). Consensus statement: a framework for safe an effective intubation by paramedics. College of Paramedics. https://collegeofparamedics.co.uk/COP/Professional_development/Intubation_Consensus_Statement_/COP/ProfessionalDevelopment/Intubation_Consensus_Statement_.aspx?hkey=5c999b6b-274b-42d3-8dbc-651c367c0493 (accessed 27 July 2020).

Cook, T., Woodall, N., and Finerk, C. (2011). NAP4: major complications of airway management in the United Kingdom. Royal College of Anaesthetists. https://www.nationalauditprojects.org.uk/NAP4_home (accessed 27 July 2020).

Frerk, C., Mitchell, V.S., McNarry, A.F. et al. (2015). Difficult Airway Society 2015 guidelines for management of unanticipated difficult intubation in adults. *British Journal of Anaesthesia* **115** (6): 827–848.

Greaves, I. and Porter, K. (2007). *Oxford Handbook of Pre-Hospital Care*. Oxford: Oxford University Press.

Gregory, P. and Mursell, I. (2010). *Manual of Clinical Paramedic Procedures*. Chichester: Wiley Blackwell.

Gregory, P. and Ward, A. (2010). *Sanders' Paramedic Textbook*. Edinburgh: Mosby Elsevier.

Pilbery, R. and Lethbridge, K. (2019). *Ambulance Care Practice*, 2e. Bridgewater: Class Professional Publishing.

Royal College of Surgeons of Edinburgh (2019). *Generic Core Material: Prehospital Emergency Care Course*. Edinburgh: Royal College of Surgeons of Edinburgh.

Needle cricothyroidotomy

Needle cricothyroidotomy is the process by which a large bore cannula is inserted into the trachea via the cricothyroid membrane as a 'last ditch' method of providing rescue oxygenation to a patient in the event of total and unmanageable airway obstruction or in the setting of can't intubate can't oxygenate (CICO). The later portion of CICO is the most important, you may be in a situation where you are unable to intubate but there are alternative methods to provide oxygenation such as supraglottic airways or simple adjuncts. Its use is predominantly is in the paediatric population as surgical airways require specific skills, exposure and training not available to the majority of pre-hospital practitioner. Adults in a CICO situation should receive a surgical airway by an appropriately trained, governed and experienced practitioner within local guidelines.

The non-technical aspect of this procedure is that the clinician will be involved in a highly stressful airway emergency. The practitioner should be aware of this and verbalise the ongoing care plan with the team as a whole before starting the procedure to ensure a shared mental model. Calling for help early with any patient with potential or actual airway compromise is paramount here.

Indications

- Rescue oxygenation for paediatrics in the event of failed airway management, including simple methods, resulting in the inability to oxygenate the patient.

Contraindications

- Absence of a suitably trained clinician in line with local policies
- Oxygenation can be provided by other simple methods
- Refer to local policies

Methodology (refer to local policy for variation)

- Indication for procedure
- **Call for help**
  - Arrange patient to receive definitive airway intervention as soon as possible
  - Pre-hospital critical care team
  - Pre-alert nearest suitable receiving unit
  - State airway emergency and that a needle cricothyroidotomy is about to be performed
- Prepare equipment including expiry date check
  - 14G cannula
  - 3-way IV extension tap with all ports open and uncapped
  - 5 mL Syringe
  - Oxygen cylinder with flow set to 1 L/min per year of age (paediatrics)
  - Tubing
    - Oxygen tubing
      OR
    - IV giving set with the chamber cut off to allow the tubing to be connected to an O_2 cylinder
  - Attach on end of the tubing to the Oxygen cylinder and the opposite end should be attached to the three-way tap connector
    - Oxygen tubing can be forced over three-way tap
    - Giving set can be screwed in place as normal
- Remove flashback chamber from cannula and attach 5 mL syringe
- Place the patient supine and in neutral alignment set yourself at the head of the patient looking down towards their toes for ease
- Prep site with wipe
- Stabilise the thyroid cartilage and identify cricothyroid membrane
- Gently but with purpose insert the needle at 45° with needle pointing towards the patients' feet
  - Aspirate the syringe during insertion
- Once the needle passes into the trachea a 'give' should be felt but, in any case, air should be aspirated easily into the syringe
- Slide the cannula off the needle into the trachea maintaining the angle as to not damage the soft posterior wall of the trachea
- Remove needle and place into sharps bin
- The cannula should be re-aspirated to confirm position
- Secure cannula in place with dressings
- Attach the 3-way tap connector as set up with oxygen attached
- Attempt to oxygenate the patient by occluding the open port of the three-way tap until the chest rises then release and allow the chest to deflate
  - Typically 1 : 4 inflation to exhalation ratio
- Transport patient to definitive airway care
  - Rendezvous with pre-hospital critical care team
  - Nearest suitable receiving unit with pre-alert provided stating clearly that a needle cricothyroidotomy has been performed and the patient has an airway obstruction

Risks

- Oesophageal puncture
- Vascular injury and bleeding
- Airway injury
- Subcutaneous placement or cannula misplacement
- Hyperinflation
- Barotrauma
- Hypercapnia

References and Further Reading

Greaves, I. and Porter, K. (2007). *Oxford Handbook of Pre-Hospital Care*. Oxford: Oxford University Press.

Gregory, P. and Mursell, I. (2010). *Manual of Clinical Paramedic Procedures*. Chichester: Wiley Blackwell.

Gregory, P. and Ward, A. (2010). *Sanders' Paramedic Textbook*. Edinburgh: Mosby Elsevier.

Royal College of Surgeons of Edinburgh (2019). *Generic Core Material: Prehospital Emergency Care Course*. Edinburgh: Royal College of Surgeons of Edinburgh.

Needle thoracocentesis

Needle thoracocentesis is the act of inserting a cannula into a patient's chest in order to relieve the pressure resulting from a tension pneumothorax. This is undertaken for patients with a deteriorating respiratory function as a result of a tension pneumothorax and not for patients who are not compromised but may have a pneumothorax. It is a technique that can be performed on spontaneously ventilating patients or in mechanically ventilated patients as a holding measure before a surgical thoracostomy is performed. Tension pneumothorax can arise as a result of trauma or from specific medical conditions such as Asthma. Developing a tension pneumothorax is also a risk when using a BVM or ventilator.

Signs of respiratory compromise secondary to tension pneumothorax are varied and may present with some or none of the following:

- Chest injury or suspicion thereof
- Breathlessness
- Hypoxia
- Tachypnoea
- Reduced air entry to affected side
  - May be subtle or overt
- Hyperresonance on affected side
  - May be difficult to elicit at noisy scenes
- Tracheal deviation
  - Difficult to stratify
  - Late sign
  - Uncommon
- Neck vein distension
  - May not be present if patient is also hypovolaemic
- Cardiac arrest

Indications

- Respiratory compromise as a result of tension pneumothorax

Contraindications

- Absence of signs consistent with tension pneumothorax
- Absence of respiratory compromise or distress

Cautions

- Thick chest wall
  - Excessive overlying muscle or fat may mean that the needle is too short to penetrate into the pleura

Methodology

- Indication for needle thoracocentesis
- Prepare equipment including expiry date check
  - 14G cannula or specific thoracocentesis cannula
  - Syringe
    - Can part fill syringe with 1–2 mL or 0.9% Sodium Chloride so that you are able to visualise bubbles if the environment is particularly noisy (RTC's etc)
  - Tape to secure
- Identify insertion site
  - 2nd intercostal space, mid-clavicular line
    OR
  - 4th/5th intercostal space mid-axillary line
  - Refer to local policy
  - Immediately above the lower rib
    - Vascular and nerve structures run underneath rubs so by going above the lower rib there is less chance of injury to these structures
- Remove flashback chamber from cannula and attach syringe
- Gently but with purpose insert the needle at 90° to the skin aspirating the syringe as you advance
- A 'give' should be felt and air aspirated into the syringe
- Pass the cannula off over the needle
- Remove the needle and place in a sharps bin
- Secure the cannula with tape
- Clearly document the procedure in the patient's notes and hand over to receiving team that the procedure has been performed

Risks

- Vascular damage
- Nerve damage
- Lung damage
- Surgical emphysema
- Cannula to short
- Cannula kinking
- Re-tension

Quick Questions

1. What are the landmarks to look for during laryngoscopy?
2. What is the indication for needle cricothyroidotomy?
3. What are the insertion sites for a needle thoracocentesis?

References and Further Reading

Greaves, I. and Porter, K. (2007). *Oxford Handbook of Pre-Hospital Care*. Oxford: Oxford University Press.
Gregory, P. and Mursell, I. (2010). *Manual of Clinical Paramedic Procedures*. Chichester: Wiley Blackwell.
Gregory, P. and Ward, A. (2010). *Sanders' Paramedic Textbook*. Edinburgh: Mosby Elsevier.
Royal College of Surgeons of Edinburgh (2019). *Generic Core Material: Prehospital Emergency Care Course*. Edinburgh: Royal College of Surgeons of Edinburgh.

169

Patient assessment

In the first section we covered some of the basics of patient assessment, this section will look to build on your knowledge and experience and give you some additional tools to help with assessing patients. Although we often discuss assessment in terms of a systems-based approach it is important to consider the patient as a whole and how one problem may be impacting on others. A firm understanding of the underlying physiology will help guide and inform your assessment. It is still important to apply a standardised approach to patients via the ABC assessment before moving on to more in-depth assessment skills. This should help you identify the 'big sick' patients who require intervention rapidly.

Scene approach

As a Paramedic or pre-hospital clinician, you have the privilege of witnessing patients at their point of presentation and not, usually, in a more clinical setting This will enable you to have a unique ability to assess the patient's surroundings as you approach them which may give you vital clues and collateral information for the assessment.

As always, the first step in approaching the scene is safety!

Additional information can be gained on approaching the patient an example of a scene approach might be:

- Is the scene safe?
- Are you safe?
- Do you need help?
  - Is there anything obvious that makes you require additional help?
  - This could be a back-up crew or specialist services such as fire and rescue, HART or HEMS.
- Access and Egress
  - Make a conscious effort to consider how you will move a patient to the ambulance if it is required as you approach
    - Size and steepness of stairs and any tight corners
    - Access through the door or alternative access
    - Can the patient be easily moved supine, if required, or will this require additional assistance?
  - Your emergency exit if required
    - Leave your personal egress route clear of obstructions including the equipment you bring with you
    - Doors unlocked or ideally open
    - Other people

- Social cues
  - The patients social setting can impact on their physical and mental health
  - As a Paramedic you will often be the only healthcare professional to see the patients social setting especially in an unaltered state
  - Are there inhalers or spray's around the patient that may indicate chronic ill-health
  - What is the state of the patient's environment?
    - Clean or cluttered
    - Cold and damp or dry and warm
    - Unusual smells
  - Ashtray or sputum pots near the patient
  - Signs of poor mobility
  - Mobility aids or rails
  - Home oxygen
  - Nebulisers
  - Signs of an unmet care need
    - Malnutrition or poor diet
    - Domestic waste removal
    - Struggling to meet activities of daily living
    - Signs of previous interactions with pre-hospital clinicians
    - Patient disclosure
  - Signs of advanced care requirements
    - Syringe drivers
    - End of life medications
    - Hospital beds
    - Home adaptations
- May be as minor as a ramp to the doorstep
- Holistic view of the patient
  - Do they comfortable in their environment
  - Are they struggling?
  - Are there any over signs that concern you?
  - Does it appear that they sleeping in their chair?
  - If they are in bed are there more pillows than would be expected

> This is not to form prejudice but to help inform a more holistic picture of the patient's environment that other clinicians later in the patient's care episode will not have easy access to

170

Greeting the patient

Your initial interaction with the patient will enable you to gather a wealth of information beyond the assessment of their 'ABC'.

As you greet the patient it may be appropriate to shake their hand, make eye contact and then ask permission to feel a radial pulse whilst you ask your initial questions and ascertain any immediate ABC considerations.

Handshake

- Are they warm or cold to touch?
- Do they feel overly hot?
- Are they clammy or diaphoretic?
- Are their hands unusually dry?
- What is the condition of their skin?
- What is the condition of their fingers?
  - Nicotine stains
  - Overtly clubbed fingers
  - Rheumatoid arthritis

Eye contact

- Colour of their sclera
  - Jaundice
  - Bloodshot
- Pallor
  - Pale
  - Jaundice
  - Cyanosed
  - Diaphoretic
- Reassuring

Radial pulse

- Present or absent
- Strong or thread
- Bounding?
- Skin turgor
- Capillary refill

ABC

- Is their airway at risk of compromise
- Is there additional effort of breathing
- Are there any immediate circulatory concerns?

Whilst the scene approach and patient greeting might seem like a lot with experience it will become second nature. It is amazing how much information can be gained from the initial parts of the assessment

Clinical questioning

- Start by asking broad and open questions, for example:
  - How can I help?
  - Do you have any pain?
  - Etc
- Use the answers from the open questions to guide relevant exploratory questions
  - 'I can't breathe'
    - For example: When did this start, have you ever had problems with your breathing before
  - 'I've got pain in my back':
    - For example: What were you doing when this started?
- This will help gain you far more information by allowing the patient to describe their condition themselves and will avoid possible confusion but jumping into an assessment
  - 'I've been getting worse for about a week now, I've got COPD'
  - 'I fell off the roof, I thought I was ok so I came inside but now I can't move'
- Once you have an idea of the presentation you can ask more focussed questions surrounding their condition or presentation

From these two very brief examples, you can see how by asking open questions you are able to allow the patient to answer open questions. The first example shows a potential chronic health condition and the second an acute trauma that otherwise could have been missed

- Questioning should never be accusatory or judgemental
- The clinician should keep an open mind throughout questioning and not try to second guess the condition
- Never try to put words into the patient's mouth, try to let them describe their condition in their own words.
- Remember to clearly document conversations and responses in the patient's notes

Respiratory assessment

- Introduction and consent
- Primary ABC assessment
    - In-depth examination should only be performed if the patient is stable and suitable for this examination
    - If the patient requires immediate intervention then this should be undertaken without delay
- Patient history

Questioning

- Onset of symptoms
    - Acute or chronic
- Duration of symptoms
- Severity
- Aggravating or alleviating factors
- Allergies or exposure to irritants
- Cough
    - Present or absent
    - If present:
        - Nature
        - Duration
        - Productivity
        - Haemoptysis
- Pain
- Fever
- Recent unexplained weight loss

Overt clinical signs

- Three E's
    - Effort
        - Is the patient having to put in additional effort in order to breathe?
    - Efficacy
        - With the effort being put in is the patient ventilating as expected?
    - Effect
        - What is the physiological result i.e. SpO_2?

Physical examination

1. Attain consent, hand hygiene, PPE as appropriate
2. Presence of tenderness and patient comfort
3. Examine the hands
    a. This differs to the initial greeting but assesses for more specific signs
        i. Cyanosis
        ii. Steroidal skin from chronic use (may be prescribed for patients with COPD)
        iii. Fine tremor (possible beta-agonist use)
        iv. Coarse tremor (assess for asterixis and CO_2 retention)

4. Examine the Neck, face and mouth
    a. Eyes
        i. Signs of anaemia which may cause shortness of breath on excursion
    b. Face
        i. Flushed or cyanotic
    c. Neck
        i. Jugular venous distension
        ii. Inflamed neck nodes
        iii. Accessory muscle use
    d. Mouth
        i. Vocal hoarseness
        ii. Pursed lips
        iii. Cyanosis
    e. Tongue
        i. Central cyanosis
        ii. Dehydration
5. Chest examination
    a. Rate
    b. Inspection (anterior and posterior)
        i. Pallor
        ii. Scars
        iii. Signs of pain
        iv. Chest shape or deformity
        v. Nutritional state
        vi. Wounds or scarring including previous burns
        vii. Symmetrical expansion
        viii. Effort of breathing

> Chest shape may affect the respiratory condition
> Funnel chest (Pectus excavatum)
> Pigeon chest (Pectus carinatum)
> Barrel chest
> Congenital conditions (kyphosis and scoliosis)

    c. Palpation (anterior and posterior)
        i. Equity in depth of respiration
        ii. Pain, tenderness, bruising, trauma, fractures
    d. Percussion (anterior and posterior)
        i. Apex to base
        ii. Equity
    e. Auscultation (anterior and posterior)
        i. Added sounds
        ii. Absent breath sounds
    f. Legs
        i. Oedema
        ii. DVT
6. Clinical observations
7. Explain findings to patient and document in the patient's notes

Cardiovascular assessment

- Introduction and consent
- Primary ABC assessment
    - In-depth examination should only be performed if the patient is stable and suitable for this examination
    - If the patient requires immediate intervention then this should be undertaken without delay
- Patient history

Questioning

- PQRST
- OLDCARTS

Overt clinical signs

- Diaphoresis
- Fist to chest
- Pallor

Physical examination

1. Attain consent, hand hygiene, PPE as appropriate
2. Presence of tenderness and patient comfort
3. Examine the hands
   a. Finger clubbing
   b. Splinter haemorrhages
   c. Signs of smoking
4. Face, eyes and tongue assessment
   a. Xanthelasma
      i. Lipid deposits normally found around the eyes but can be present over whole body
      ii. Sign of hyperlipidaemia
   b. Corneal arcus
      i. 'Whitish ring' surrounding the iris
      ii. Also, a sign of hyperlipidaemia
   c. Anaemia
   d. Jugular venous distension
5. Examine the chest for scars indicating previous surgery
   a. Mid-line sternotomy
   b. Left thoracotomy scar
   c. Pacemaker or implantable defibrillation device scar
6. Peripheral pitting oedema
   a. Dependant oedema i.e. ankles
   b. Sacral oedema
7. Pulse
   a. Assess for rate, rhythm and regularity
8. Capillary refill time
   a. Suggestive of peripheral perfusion
   b. Skin turgor testing can be done simultaneously
9. Heart sounds
   a. Heart sounds originate from the **closure** of heart valves
   b. S1 and S2 sounds
      i. S1 indicates the closure of Atrioventricular valves and the beginning of systole
      ii. S2 indicates the closure of semilunar valves at diastole
   c. Third heart sound or S3
      i. Normal finding in children, young adults and during pregnancy
      ii. May be pathological in patients aged over 40 commonly suggesting left ventricular failure and/or mitral regurgitation

     d. Murmur
        i. Produced by turbulent blood flow across an abnormal valve
        ii. If it doesn't sound completely normal then it should be investigate further
     e. Muffled heart sounds
        i. Obesity
        ii. Fluid in the pericardial sac (cardiac effusion or tamponade)
     f. Pericardial friction rub
        i. Scratching, grating or squeaking quality
        ii. Associated with pericarditis

10. Bruits

     a. Abnormal sound heard during auscultation of carotid artery (can be heard elsewhere)
     b. May indicate local obstruction
     c. Auscultate carotid artery using the bell of the stethoscope asking the patient to hold their breath

11. Tactile thrills
     a. Similar to bruits normally detected as fine vibration or tremors
     b. Suggest interference with blood flow
     c. May be palatable above the site of an aneurism

12. Baseline observations

13. Concurrent respiratory examination is helpful

14. ECG 12 lead

15. Explain findings to patient and document in the patient's notes

Neurological examination

Neurological examination encompasses three main areas; higher cerebral functions, central nervous system functions, cerebellar function and the peripheral nervous system. Although, a dysfunction with one system may manifest in the examination of another.

- Introduction and consent
- Primary ABC assessment
  - In-depth examination should only be performed if the patient is stable and suitable for this examination
  - If the patient requires immediate intervention then this should be undertaken without delay
- Patient history

Questioning

- Sensation changes
  - Numbness, paraesthesia, smell
- Headaches, faints, dizziness
- Thought processing, memory and speech disturbances
- Pain
- Bladder and/or bowel dysfunction
- Issues with swallowing

Overt clinical signs

- Facial droop
- Speech disturbances
- Unilateral weakness
- Coma/reduced level of consciousness

Physical examination

1. Attain consent, hand hygiene, PPE as appropriate
2. Presence of tenderness and patient comfort
3. Higher cerebral functions
   a. Glasgow Coma Score
   b. Mini-Mental State Exam
   c. Speech and thought processing
4. Central nervous system
   a. Cranial nerves exam
5. Cerebellar function
6. Peripheral nervous system
7. Explain findings to patient and document in the patient's notes

Cranial nerves

1. Olfactory
2. Optic
3. Oculomotor
4. Trochlear
5. Trigeminal
6. Abducens
7. Facial
8. Vestibulocochlear
9. Glossopharyngeal
10. Vagus
11. Accessory
12. Hypoglossal

Many pneuonics are available to help remember the cranial nerves try and find one that works for you.

Testing the cranial nerves

- General overview
  - GCS
  - Facial symmetry
- Snellens chart
  - May not be available pre-hospital
  - Use surroundings i.e. posters or newspapers
- Visual fields
  - High and low
- Pupil inspection
  - Shape
  - Abnormalities
- Pupil reaction
  - Direct
  - Consensual
- Near-Far response
  - Accommodation
  - Convergence
- 'H' gaze
  - Trace the shape of an 'H' with your finger
  - Check the eyes follow in every plane of movement

- Nystagmus
  - Follow your finger as you rapidly bring it horizontally to the extreme of visual field
  - Observe for eye flickering
- Facial sensation
  - Crude
  - Sharp/dull differentiation
- Temporal and masseter muscles
  - Inspect
  - Palpate
- Facial movements
  - Smile
  - Frown
  - Puff cheeks out
- Whisper test
  - Stand behind patient
  - Rub fingers together beside ear and ask patient which ear they can hear it in
- Throat
  - Say 'Ahhh'
  - Watch uvula to check stays in the midline
- Shoulder shrug
  - Active and resisted
- Head turn
  - Active and resisted
- Tongue out
  - In the midline?
- Phonation
  - 'Right, Tight, Dynamite'
  - 'Baby Hippopotamus'

Testing the peripheral nervous system

- General overview
- Tone
  - Upper
  - Lower
- Clonus
  - Ankle
- Strength
  - Grip
  - Bicep/Tricep
  - Shoulder
  - Hip flexion and extension
  - Knee flexion and extension
- Reflexes
  - Not commonly performed pre-hospital
  - If suitably trained
- Sensory
  - Sharp vs dull sensation
- Proprioception
  - Thumb up/down movements with eyes closed

- Coordination
  - Hold out your finger
  - Ask patient to touch your finger with theirs and then touch their nose
  - Move finger across midline and repeat
  - Repeat with both arms
- Localisation
  - Eyes closed
  - Touch forearm of ankle and ask patient to touch the same place
- Heel to shin
  - Both sides
- Dysdiadochokinesis
  - 'Flip flop' one hand on top of the other
- Romberg test
  - Safe position
  - Eyes closed and feet together
  - Observe for swaying
  - Be ready to catch patient or tell to open eyes
- Pronator drift
  - Arms out in front, palms up
  - Eyes closed
  - Observe if one arm drifts without input
  - Can tap one hand then the other and ask patient to keep where they are
- Gait (if normally mobile enough)
  - Normal
  - Walking on heels
  - Walking on toes
  - Heel-to-toe (if mobile enough)

Abdominal assessment

- Introduction and consent
- Primary ABC assessment
  - In-depth examination should only be performed if the patient is stable and suitable for this examination
  - If the patient requires immediate intervention then this should be undertaken without delay
- Patient history

Questioning

- Pain
  - PQRST
  - OLDCARTS
- Change in bowel habits
- Appetite and/or weight loss
- Change in urine including pain on passing

Overt clinical signs

- Bruising
- Pulsatile masses
- Vomiting

- Hematemesis
- PR/PV/PU bleeding
- Scars
- Catheters

Physical examination

1. Attain consent, hand hygiene, PPE as appropriate
2. Presence of tenderness and patient comfort
3. General overview
   a. Pallor
   b. Abdomen size, shape, distension
   c. General health
4. Examine the patient's hands
   a. Palmar erythema
   b. Clubbing
   c. Nail condition
   d. Tremor
   e. Liver flap
5. Examine the patient's face
   a. Sclera for jaundice
   b. Conjunctiva
   c. Mouth and dentition
6. Examine the patient's neck
   a. Lymph nodes
   b. Take note of left-sided clavicular nodes if raised
7. Lie the patient flat, expose as appropriate and with consent
   a. Ensure patient dignity
   b. Chaperones
8. Inspect the abdomen
   a. Contours
   b. Symmetry
   c. Umbilicus
   d. Hair
   e. Spider Naevi
   f. Hernias
   g. Stomas
   h. Caput medusa
9. Auscultate
   a. Bowel sounds
10. Percussion
    a. Dull
    b. Tympany
    c. Fluid shift
11. Palpation
    a. Light then deep
    b. Pulses
    c. Liver
    d. Spleen
    e. Tenderness
    f. On palpation or relief (rebound)

12. Costovertebral angle tenderness (renal)
13. Ask about genital pain, discharge and discomfort
14. Explain findings to patient and document in the patient's notes

Additional abdominal signs

- Rovsing's sign
  - Palpating the RIGHT iliac fossa may illicit pain in the LEFT
  - Indicative of Appendicitis
- Murphy's sign
  - Deep palpation RIGHT mid-clavicular line directly below the rib cage
  - Patient takes a deep breath in
  - Pain worsens as gallbladder descends onto palpating hand
  - Indicative of cholecystitis or biliary colic

References and Further Reading

Bickley, L.S. (2013). *Bates' Guide to Physical Examination and History Taking*, 11e. Philidelphia: Wolters Kluwer.

Douglas, G., Nicol, F., and Robertson, C. (2013). *Macleod's Clinical Examination*, 13e. Edinburgh: Churchill Livingstone Elsevier.

Greaves, I. and Porter, K. (2007). *Oxford Handbook of Pre-Hospital Care*. Oxford: Oxford University Press.

Gregory, P. and Ward, A. (2010). *Sanders' Paramedic Textbook*. Edinburgh: Mosby Elsevier.

Hammond, B.B. and Zimmermann, P.G. (2013). *Sheehy's Manual of Emergency Care*, 7e. Missouri: Mosby.

OME (2019). Mini-mental state examination. http://www.oxfordmedicaleducation.com/geriatrics/mini-mental-state-examination-mmse/ (accessed 30 October 2020).

Pilbery, R. and Lethbridge, K. (2019). *Ambulance Care Practice*, 2e. Bridgewater: Class Professional Publishing.

Raftery, A.T., Lim, E., and Ostor, A.J.K. (2014). *Churchill's Pocketbook of Differential Diagnosis*, 4e. Edinburgh: Churchill Livingstone Elsevier.

Royal College of Surgeons of Edinburgh (2019). *Generic Core Material: Prehospital Emergency Care Course*. Edinburgh: Royal College of Surgeons of Edinburgh.

Rushforth, H. (2009). *Assessment Made Incredibly Easy!* Philidelphia: Wolters Kluwer.

The 12 lead ECG

The 12 lead ECG provides a 2-Dimensional representation of the 3-Dimensional structure of the heart. It utilised the four limb leads and six chest leads to acquire a tracing of the heart for interpretation.

It is important for the Paramedic to recognise their limitations with ECG interpretation, Doctors who specialise in Cardiology will undergo many years specific training to identify minor abnormalities in the ECG, you will not be expected to interpret and ECG to the same level. As a Paramedic it is important to recognise four main domains of ECG's.

1. The normal ECG
   a. An ECG that does not require further investigation
2. The abnormal ECG that requires primary percutaneous intervention
   a. An ECG that shows changes consistent with acute myocardial infarction
3. The abnormal ECG but does not require primary intervention
   a. An ECG not indicative of MI but requires further investigation, treatment or referral
4. The emergency ECG
   a. An ECG that requires immediate defibrillation or CPR

These four domains build on the premise of: 'if in doubt – refer'. If you are able to spot an abnormality but not quantify it should be referred to a specialist.

The ECG is a single aspect of the cardiovascular assessment and should be interpreted along with the patient's physiological findings. Some patients may present with extremely abnormal ECG's but their physiology is not affected. Remember to treat the patient first.

Cardiology is a subspecialty of medicine that a doctor will train for 8+ years to become an expert in. You are not expected as a paramedic to operate at the same level, do not feel disheartened if you can't identify every subtle ECG change but focus on the four domains as mentioned above and treating the patient as a whole not just their ECG.

Normal intervals

PR interval = 0.12–0.2 seconds
QRS interval = 0.08–0.12 seconds
QT interval = 0.35–0.45 seconds

Placement of the chest leads

Table 8.2   Position of the chest leads.

V1	4th intercostal space RIGHT sternal margin
V2	4th intercostal space LEFT sternal margin
V3	Midway between V2 and V4 (to be placed after V4)
V4	5th intercostal space LEFT mid-clavicular line
V5	5th intercostal space LEFT anterior axillary line
V6	5th intercostal space LEFT mid-axillary line

There may be occasions whereby you have to move the ECG leads because of the rhythm shown. This may be for a possible right-sided MI or posterior involvement.
Right-sided

Table 8.3   Placement of right-sided ECG.

V4r	5th intercostal space RIGHT mid-clavicular line

If an MI is suspected then you should not delay treatment and transport to perform these unless clinically indicated. If performed the ECG should be clearly annotated with the lead position to avoid confusion

Posterior

Table 8.4   Placement of a posterior ECG.

V7	LEFT posterior axillary line at level of V6
V8	Tip of LEFT scapula level with V7
V9	LEFT paraspinal region level with V7

Regions of the heart

The ECG leads will correspond to areas of the heart and changes may indicate damage to a specific area. This will help you understand the physiology you may then see.

Table 8.5 Depicting the regions affected if there is associated ST segment changes.

I		AVr		V1		V4	
	Lateral				Septal		Anterior
II		AVl		V2		V5	
	Inferior		Lateral		Septal		Lateral
III		AVf		V3		V6	
	Inferior		Inferior		Anterior		Lateral

A helpful way to remember these is: 'Liar Liar Say All'			
L		S	A
I	L	S	L
I	I	A	L

Vascular supply to the heart

As well as understanding the regions you can then consider the ECG in terms of which vessel may be affected in acute MI.

Table 8.6 Rough correlation between areas of ST segment changes and coronary vessel lesion.

I		AVr		V1		V4	
	Circumflex				LAD		
II		AVl		V2		V5	
	RCA		Circumflex		LAD		Circumflex
III		AVf		V3		V6	
	RCA		RCA				Circumflex

An approach to ECG interpretation

1. Begin by assessing the 3-lead rhythm strip
2. Is there any electrical activity?
3. What is the ventricular (QRS) rate?

4. Is the QRS rhythm regular or irregular
5. Is the QRS with normal or widened?
6. Is there atrial activity?
7. Is every P wave followed by a QRS?
8. Does every QRS have a P wave before it?
9. Determine the rhythm and cardiac axis
    a. Normal axis – Leads I and aVF will be positive
    b. Left axis – Lead I is positive. aVF will be negative
        i. This will appear as they are '<u>L</u>eaving' the page
    c. Right axis – Lead I will be negative. aVF will be positive
        i. They will appear to '<u>R</u>each' towards each other
10. Exclude possible pre-excitation
    a. PR interval of less than 0.12 seconds (three small squares)
11. Exclude atrioventricular blocks
    a. PR interval of greater than 0.2 seconds (five small squares)
12. Exclude left bundle branch block
13. Exclude right bundle branch block
14. Assess the chest leads
    a. ST segment abnormalities
    b. Any other abnormalities
15. Look at the limb leads
    a. ST segment abnormalities
    b. Any other abnormalities
16. Explain findings to patient and document in the patient's notes

References and Further Reading

Gregory, P. and Mursell, I. (2010). *Manual of Clinical Paramedic Procedures.* Chichester: Wiley Blackwell.

Gregory, P. and Ward, A. (2010). *Sanders' Paramedic Textbook.* Edinburgh: Mosby Elsevier.

Hampton, J. and Hampton, J. (2019). *The ECG Made Easy*, 9e. Edinburgh: Elsevier.

Herring, N. and Paterson, D.J. (2018). *Levick's Introduction to Cardiovascular Physiology*, 6e. London: CRC Press.

Life In The Fast Lane (2021). https://litfl.com/ecg-library/basics.

Pilbery, R. and Lethbridge, K. (2019). *Ambulance Care Practice*, 2e. Bridgewater: Class Professional Publishing.

Tortora, G.J. and Derrickson, B.H. (2017). *Tortora's Principles of Anatomy and Physiology*, 15e. Chichester: Wiley.

9

Pharmacology – 2

Contents

In the first section, we covered the basics of pharmacokinetics and pharmacodynamics as well as looking at the administration of medicines. This section will look to build on your knowledge surrounding pharmacology.

Cell signalling

Cell signally describes the process whereby information is shared between cells to maintain homeostasis.

- Cells within the body are 'talking' to each other constantly
- This is done by the release of chemicals from the cell
  - Majority of signalling is done by cytokines
  - Cytokines is a general term encompassing a wide array of small proteins
- These chemicals can affect the same cell, neighbouring cells or cells elsewhere in the body
- Without these signals, the cell is programmed to 'self destruct' in a process known as apoptosis
- Cell signalling can be a target for medications

There are three main types of cell signalling.

- Autocrine
  - Cell 'talking' to itself
- Paracrine
  - Cell 'talking' locally i.e. neighbouring cells
- Endocrine
  - Cells 'talking' distantly

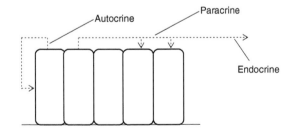

Figure 9.1 Depicting cell signalling.

Cell signalling is used in the maintenance of homeostasis and cell monitoring. If a cell begins to behave 'strangely', this will result in an altered cell signalling.

The Paramedic Revision Guide, First Edition. David W. Thom.
© 2021 John Wiley & Sons Ltd. Published 2021 by John Wiley & Sons Ltd.

For example, if a liver cell began emitting cytokines associated with another type of cell such as an ovary.

- Incorrect cytokines released in the paracrine messaging
- Neighbouring cells release 'S.O.S.' cytokines
- Killer T Cells activated by the SOS cytokines
- Killer T Cells 'assess' the faulty cell
- If faulty the cells will express a glycoprotein on their not that is not recognised as being 'normal' for the cell
- Cell destroyed by killer T cells

Cytokines

- Cytokines act as 'Morse code' for cell signalling
- Small proteins are released in a specific order to create a chemical message
    - Right order = message conveyed and appropriate actions
    - Wrong order = wrong message

If a cell begins emitting the wrong cytokine order or stops emitting cytokines altogether, this will be 'sensed' by the neighbouring cells.

- Wrong order
    - Wrong effect
    - No effect
    - Cell death (apoptosis)
- No signals
    - Cell death (apoptosis)

So why is this important? Cell signalling or disorders of signalling can result in the pathology you encounter as a paramedic but it can also be 'interfered with' with medications.

In the first section, we covered the RICE acronym for target sites of medications. This section will look to build on your knowledge and add a bit more detail.

Receptors

Receptors are innervated by a substrate to form a reaction.
There are four main categories of receptors.

- Inotropic (ligand gated)
- Metabotropic (G-Coupled)
- Kinase linked (enzyme linked)
- Nuclear

Ionotropic

- Usually have four trans-membrane domains (TMD)
- TMD's are target sites for drugs
- TMD's cross the cell membrane and enable a drug to exert it's effect by causing a reaction within the cell
- Sometimes have five TMD's
- Means both N and C terminals sit outside cell membrane if 4TMD therefore more binding sites
- Example
    - Nicotinic Receptor
        - Innervated by Acetyl-Choline (Ach), Gamma-Aminobutyric Acid ($GABA_A$), serotonin ($5HT_3$)

G-Coupled

- Seven TMD's
- Four target enzymes
  - Guanylate cyclase
  - Adenylate cyclase
  - Phospholipase C
  - Phospholipase A_2 – note role in inflammation
- Five secondary messengers
  - cGMP (c-Guanosine Mono-Phosphate)
  - cAMP (c-Adenosine Mono-Phosphate)
  - IP_3 – Inocytylphosphate
    - Specifically alter CA^{2+} levels
  - DAG (diglyceride)
  - AA (Arachidonic Acid)
- Examples
  - Muscurinic Ach (mAChR)
  - Adrenoreceptors (α and β)
  - Dopamine receptors
  - Opioid receptors
  - 5HT receptors
    - Not $5HT_3$
  - Purine (Caffeine and adenosine)
  - Receptors in special senses (smell/sight/taste)

Kinase-linked receptors

- Involve tyrosine-kinase and guanylate cyclase
- Two pathways
  - Ras/Raf/MAP kinase = cell division and growth
  - Jak/Stat = cytokines and inflammation
- Examples
  - Insulin
  - Growth hormone
  - Cytokines

Nuclear

- Regulate DNA transcription and protein expression
- Powerful
- Slow as have to cross cell membrane and nuclear membrane
- Examples include
  - Steroid receptors
  - Thyroid hormone receptors
  - Vitamin D
  - Retinoic acid

Ion channels

- Provides a rapid response to signal
- Rapid response vital to
  - Central nervous system
  - Cardiovascular system
  - Renal system
- Innervated by a ligand which is equivalent of a substrate for a receptor

Carrier molecules

- The movement of substances across the cell membrane often requires a carrier molecule.
- Carrier molecules are usually for
  - Ions
  - Glucose
  - Amino acids
  - Large molecules.
- Examples
  - Sodium Potassium pump
    - Uses sodium potassium ATP-ase as an enzyme to drive the Na^+/K^+ pump

Enzymes

An enzyme is a protein (or protein based molecule) that acts as a catalyst to speed up a chemical reaction. An enzyme acts on specific substances known as substrates.
   Drug/Enzyme interactions may involve

- Substrate analogues
  - Similar to i.e. the drug is similar to normal substrate
  - Reversible inhibitors bind to enzyme via weak NON-covalent bonds (i.e. hydrogen/ionic bonds) and can be easily removed.
  - These bonds are fairly non-specific.
- False substrates
  - Drug almost identical to normal substrate
  - Drug molecule behaves like normal substrate and is acted upon by the enzyme to produce an ABNORMAL product that disrupts the normal pathway.
    - Products usually inactive therefore stops the pathway
- Conversion of pro-drugs
  - The drug is not in active form when administered
  - Enzyme converts substrate in to active form
  - Example
    - Codeine is converted into morphine by enzymes
- Can't guarantee therapeutic or toxic levels as cannot guarantee effectiveness of enzymes especially in children and the elderly
    - ACE inhibitors
- Most are inactive in tablet form but are converted into their active metabolites

Pharmacology of the nervous system

Ganglions

- A ganglion is a neuronal cell body that sits outside of the central nervous system
- Synapse between myelinated pre-ganglionic fibres and non-myelinated post-ganglionic fibres
- Allows for the change in neurotransmitters
  - Neurotransmitter at ganglion is acetylcholine (ACh)
  - Post-ganglionic (affector) neurotransmitters differ between sympathetic and parasympathetic
    - Sympathetic will use Norepinephrine
    - Parasympathetic will use ACh

Parasympathetic nervous system

- Arises from cell bodies of cranial nerves III, VII, IX and X in brain stem and the 2nd, 3rd and 4th segments of sacral spinal cord
- Conservation and restoration of energy
- Long pre-ganglionic fibres, short post-ganglionic fibre
- Neurotransmitter is ACh
- Nicotinic and muscarinic receptors
  - Nicotinic = Ionic receptor
  - Muscurinic = G-Coupled protein receptor

Sympathetic nervous system

- Arises from cell bodies lateral to gray horns of spinal cord from the 1st thoracic to 2nd lumbar segments
- Rapid mobilisation of energy
- Spinal ganglia down the side of the spine
- Short pre-ganglionic fibres and long post-ganglionic fibres
- Uses ACh pre-ganglionic and noradrenaline post-ganglionic
- Uses α and β receptors
  - Both are G-coupled protein receptors

> ### Quick summary
>
> - Autonomic Nervous System responsible for maintaining homeostasis
> - Involuntary control
> - Two divisions
>   - Sympathetic and parasympathetic
> - Anatomical and functional differences
> - ACh used throughout parasympathetic
> - ACh used pre-ganglionic and NorAd used post-ganglionic in sympathetic
> - Nicotinic and muscarinic in parasympathetic
> - Alpha and beta in sympathetic

Nicotinic receptors

- Nicotinic ACh receptors ('nAChR')
- ACh is the ligand
- Coupled to cat-ion channels (allows passage of +ve charged ions)
- Membrane depolarisation and fast excitatory transmission
- Two subtypes
  - Muscle type
  - Neuronal type

> Nicotinic receptors utilise Ach a the ligand and not nicotine as you might expect.

- Agonists
  - ACh
  - Nicotine
- Antagonists
  - Muscular blockers
- ACh binds to the α subunit which causes change in shape and ion channel to open

Muscarinic receptors

- 'mAChR'
- ACh is the ligand
- G-coupled protein receptors
- Three main subtypes
  - M1 – Neural
  - M2 – Cardiac
  - M3 – Smooth muscle
- Agonists examples
  - Carbachol
  - Bethanechol
- Antagonists examples
  - Atropine
  - Ipratropium

Anticholinesterase drugs

- ACh is broken down by cholinesterase
- Drugs inhibiting this temporarily boost ACh levels at synapse
- Therefore they increase the expected effects of ACh at that level

Adrenoceptors

- α has two subtypes α1 and α2
  - α1 – vasoconstriction
  - α2 – vascular smooth muscle
- β has three subtypes β1, β2 and β3
  - β1 – cardiac
  - β2 – Airways (smooth muscle)
  - β3 – lipolysis and neutrophils
    - Found in adipose tissues and neonates

So why is this important? Lets look at some examples of drugs you might use in your practice.

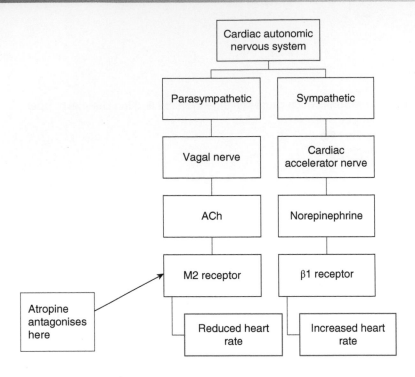

Figure 9.2   Cardiac nervous system and drugs.

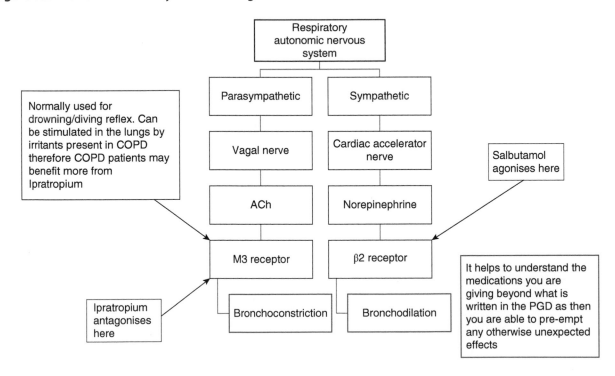

Figure 9.3   Respiratory nervous system and drugs.

Pain

Pain is 'an unpleasant sensory and emotional experience associated with actual or potential tissue damage or described in terms of such damage' (Merskey 1979).
Pain is:

- Transmitted through dorsal horn of spinal cord
  - Synapses in spinal cord are the 'gates'
- Neuropeptides
  - Glutamate = excitatory
  - GABA = inhibitory
- A and C fibres
  - A-delta fibres are fast myelinated fibres
  - Sharp pain
  - C fibres are slow non-myelinated
  - Dull pain
- Centrally modulated
- Descending inhibitory neurotransmitters are
  - 5HT
  - Endorphins
  - Enkephalins
  - Noradrenaline

Tissue damage

- Tissue injury releases phospholipid
- Phospholipid broken down by Phospholipase A2 into Arachadonic Acid
- Arachadonic acid is secondary messenger
- Arachadonic acid innervates two pathways
  - Cyclooxygenase (COX) pathway (COX-1, COX-2, and COX-3)
    - Activate prostaglandins
  - Lipoxygenase
    - Activate Leukotriene's

Prostaglandins

- Some are needed for normal function
- Mainly PGE2
  - PGE2 also active in stomach lining for protection
  - Responsible for renal blood flow
    - Reduced PGE2 = reduced renal blood flow
- Also interact with Thromboxane A2

Opioid receptors

- Mu responsible for most analgesic effects and common side effects
  - I.e. respiratory depression

- All opioid receptors G-protein linked
- Open K$^+$ channels and block Ca^{2+} channels.

Pharmacology of analgesia

Non-Steroidal Anti-Inflammatories (NSAID's)

- Most are weak acids
- Absorption from stomach and small intestine
- Highly protein bound
- Hepatic metabolism
    - Some enterohepatic circulation
- Usually work by blocking the COX pathway
- By blocking COX pathway this will up-regulate the leukotriene production as the Arachadonic Acid can only innervate the Lipoxygenase pathway
    - Responsible for irritation in asthma and bronchospasm
- Side effects related to normal physiological role of prostaglandins
    - GI bleed
    - Hypersensitivity reactions
    - Renal damage
    - Impairment of blood clotting
    - Liver damage

Mild opioids

- Include morphine analogues
    - Codeine/dihydrocodeine
- Synthetic derivatives of morphine
- Work by weakly agonising opioid receptors
    - Found on inhibitory pathways
- Codeine
    - No increased effect with increased dose
    - Genetic pre-disposition to converting enzymes
- Tramadol
    - Inhibits 5HT and noradrenaline re-uptake

Strong opioids

- Morphine analogues
    - Morphine
    - Diamorphine
    - High affinity for mu receptors
- Synthetic derivatives
    - Fentanyl
    - Oxycodone
- Morphine has significant 1st pass effect
    - Converted in the liver to active metabolites

References and Further Reading

Merskey, H. (1979). Pain terms: a list with definitions and notes on usage. Recommended by the IASP subcommittee on taxonomy. *Pain* **6**: 249–252.

Nutall, D. and Rutt-Howard, J. (2019). *The Textbook of Non-Medical Prescribing*, 3e. Chichester: Wiley Blackwell.

Ritter, J.M., Flower, R.J., Henderson, G. et al. (2019). *Rang and Dale's Pharmacology*, 9e. Edinburgh: Elsevier.

Tortora, G.J. and Derrickson, B.H. (2017). *Tortora's Principles of Anatomy and Physiology*, 15e. Chichester: Wiley.

Treede, R.-F. (2018). The international association for the study of pain definition of pain: as valid in 2018 as in 1979, but in need of regularly updated footnotes. *Pain Reports* **3** (2): e643.

Waugh, A. and Grant, A. (2018). *Ross and Wilson Anatomy and Physiology*. Edinburgh: Elsevier.

Whalen, K. (2018). *Pharmacology*, 7e. Philidelphia: Wolters Kluwer.

10

Medical emergencies – 2

Contents

This section will look to add a few more conditions to what has been covered already in section one.

Hyperglycaemia

Presentation

- Raised blood sugar
- Dehydration
- Kussmaul's respirations
- Tachycardia
- Confusion/agitation
- Lethargy
- Emesis (vomiting)
- Coma may be present

Pathophysiology

- Relative or absolute lack of insulin
- Inability to process sugar through normal routes
- Rise in blood glucose
- Raised plasma glucose levels causes increased urine glucose and osmotic diuresis
- Mobilisation of fatty acid from stores
- Fatty acids metabolised in the liver by ketogenesis
- Resultant metabolic acidaemia

The Paramedic Revision Guide, First Edition. David W. Thom.
© 2021 John Wiley & Sons Ltd. Published 2021 by John Wiley & Sons Ltd.

Treatment

- Maintain airway patency
- High flow oxygen therapy
  - Acidaemia will cause shift in oxygen disassociation
- Fluid therapy in line with local policy
- Immediate transfer to hospital for specialist treatment

Specific considerations

- May be a sign of underlying infection
- In children may be a first presentation of diabetes
- Hyperglycaemia with acidosis is a complex physiological condition requiring specific treatment in hospital
- Over infusion of crystalloid may have profound physiological effects, note that dehydration is a side effect and the mainstay of treatment is 'turning off' the ketosis by the patient receiving specific insulin infusions in hospital

195

Pulmonary embolus

Presentation

- Dependant of degree of obstruction
- Chest pain
- Shortness of breath
- Hypoxia
- Tachypnoea
- Tachycardia
- Syncope
- Massive PE
  - Hypotension < 90 mmHg
- Sub-massive PE
  - Signs of Right Ventricular failure or myocardial necrosis but *without* hypotension
- Non-massive PE
  - Signs of PE but without severe features as noted above

Pathophysiology

- Thrombus within the arterial tree
  - Usually from a Deep Vein Thrombosis elsewhere in the body
- Thrombus restricts blood flow through the pulmonary circulation
- Reduced blood flow to areas of the lung where ventilation is occurring
  - Less surface area being perfused
  - Less opportunity for oxygen to diffuse into the circulation
  - The phenomenon of ventilating a section of lung that is not being perfused can be referred to as a shunt
  - There is a difference or 'mismatch' between the Ventilation (V) and Perfusion (handily denoted as Q)
  - Referred to as a V/Q mismatch
- Restriction in the outflow from the right side of the heart can lead to right ventricular strain
- Reduced blood flow though the pulmonary circulation will result in a reduced pre-load to the left side of the heart and therefore reduced systemic circulation and features of left ventricular failure i.e. syncope and hypotension

Treatment

- High flow oxygen therapy
- Emergency admission to hospital
- Fluid as per local policy

Special considerations

- S1, Q3, T3 is a rare finding and should not be relied upon for determining PE

Acute left ventricular failure with pulmonary oedema

Presentation

- Shortness of breath
- Tachypnoea
- Tachycardia
- 'Bubbling' sounds
- Coarse crepitations on auscultation
- Hypoxia
- Fear/Panic

Pathophysiology

- Damaged or failing left ventricle
- Ventricle is unable to generate sufficient pressure to overcome the afterload
- Reduced cardiac output as stroke volume becomes reduced
- As the left ventricle is unable to fully eject the blood there is a 'backlog' within the pulmonary circulation
- Increased intra-vascular pressure within the pulmonary circulation causes fluid shift out of the vessels into the alveoli
- Build up of fluid within the alveoli making gas exchange difficult and reduced oxygen delivery to the vessels and ultimately the tissues
- Hypoxic blood and poor filling of the coronary arteries worsens cardiac failure

Treatment

- Oxygen therapy
  - Increases available oxygen
  - Increases the partial pressure to steepen the gradient across the fluid layer in the alveoli
- Nitrates
  - Vasodilatation to reduce afterload and encourage forward flow from the heart
  - As per local policy
- Furosemide
  - Diuresis to reduce pre-load
  - Some vasodilator effects
  - Slow onset
  - As per local policy

- Continuous Positive Airway Pressure (CPAP)
  - May be available through local critical care services

Specific considerations

- Left ventricular failure is only one cause of pulmonary oedema
- Failing hearts will continue to fail unless acted upon

Hypothermia

Presentation

- Mild (32–35 °C)
  - Shivering
  - Reduced co-ordination
  - Discomfort
  - Raised heart rate, blood pressure and respiratory rate
- Moderate (30–32 °C)
  - Muscle rigidity
  - Confusion
  - Slow and/or slurred speech
  - Reduced blood pressure
  - Arrhythmia
- Severe (<30 °C)
  - Exhaustion
  - Weakness
  - Drunk like appearance
  - Unconsciousness/coma
  - Bradycardia and/or arrhythmia's degrading into VF
  - Slow or absent respiration
  - Severe hypotension making it difficult to feel a pulse

> Unconscious hypothermic patients may appear dead without a pulse or breathing but may be successfully resuscitated given the right circumstances and treatment.

Pathophysiology

- Body is able to compensate for small shifts in core temperature but if the environment is such that it exceeds the bodies ability the core temperature may drop
- Acute hypothermia is rapid onset such as falling into ice water
- Sub-acute hypothermia occurs over a greater period of time such as walker/climbers without proper protective equipment
- Onset can be insidious and nay go unnoticed especially if effecting a whole group at once
- Metabolic demand decreases with core temperature

Treatment

- Mild
  - Consider specialist help
  - Move the patient to warm and dry shelter
  - Reduce further heat loss by adding dry blankets

- Moderate
  - Seek specialist help
  - Move the patient to warm and dry shelter
  - Gently warm the patient as able
  - Warming may take some time
- Severe
  - Seek specialist help
  - Carefully move the patient to warm and dry shelter
  - Remove any wet clothing and replace with dry blankets
  - Cover the patients head
  - Avoid any unnecessary movement as this may precipitate cardiac arrest
  - Avoid placing the patient upright
  - Avoid rapid re-warming
- Cardiac arrest
  - If core temp <30 °C then no more than 3 shocks should be given until the temperature is above 30 °C
  - If core temp <30 °C then withhold resuscitation drugs as they are likely to be ineffective
  - Once above 30 °C then drugs could be given with the interval doubled (i.e. every 8–10 minutes)
    - This is due to altered metabolism of the drugs
  - Chest compressions and ventilation may be more difficult
  - A hypothermic patient cannot be declared dead until re-warmed
  - Multiple options for re-warming are available within the hospital
  - Hypothermia despite being a reversible cause is neuroprotective

> Temperature should be taken by an oesophageal temperature probe for a core temperature when able. Critical care teams may have these.

Special considerations

- Consider your personal safety if you are in an environment that lead to a patient becoming hypothermic
- Seek specialist advice and assistance early
- Moving severely hypothermic patients may precipitate cardiac arrest

Questions

1. True or false
   a. Kussmaul's respirations are typically associated with hypoglycaemia
   b. Massive PE presents with a systolic blood pressure of <90 mmHg
   c. Nitrates can be used to treat pulmonary oedema.
2. What might you expect to see in a patient with moderate hypothermia.
3. How might you treat hyperglycaemia?

References and Further Reading

Association of Ambulance Chief Executives (2019). *JRCALC Clinical Guidelines*. Bridgewater: Class Professional Publishing.

Bersten, A.D. and Handy, J.M. (2018). *Oh's Intensive Care Manual*. Edinburgh: Elsevier.

Bourke, S.J. and Burns, G.P. (2015). *Respiratory Medicine: Lecture Notes*, 9e. Chichester: Wiley Blackwell.

Farkas, J. (2016). The Internet book of critical care. EMCrit. https://emcrit.org/ibcc/toc/ (accessed 21 July 2020).

Greaves, I. and Porter, K. (2007). *Oxford Handbook of Pre-Hospital Care*. Oxford: Oxford University Press.

Gregory, P. and Ward, A. (2010). *Sanders' Paramedic Textbook*. Edinburgh: Mosby Elsevier.

Harris, T. and Jones J.M. (2018). Cardiac arrest in special circumstances: hypothermic cardiac arrest. Royal College of Emergency Medicine. https://www.rcemlearning.co.uk/reference/cardiac-arrest-in-special-circumstances-hypothermic-cardiac-arrest/#1568299302640-2e315b45-a32e (accessed 12 August 2020).

Heaton, T. (2020). The Gasman handbook. http://www.thegasmanhandbook.co.uk (accessed 6 August 2020).

Kaufman, D.P., Kandle, P.F., Murray, I. et al. (2020). Physiology, oxyhemoglobin disassociation curve. StatPearls. https://www.ncbi.nlm.nih.gov/books/NBK499818/ (accessed 6 August 2020).

Nickson, C. (2019). Ketoacidosis. LITFL. https://litfl.com/ketoacidosis/ (accessed 6 August 2020).

Norris, T.L. (2018). *Porth's Pathophysiology: Concepts of Altered Health States*, 10e. Philidelphia: Wolters Kluwer.

Royal College of Surgeons of Edinburgh (2019). *Generic Core Material: Prehospital Emergency Care Course*. Edinburgh: Royal College of Surgeons of Edinburgh.

Tortora, G.J. and Derrickson, B.H. (2017). *Tortora's Principles of Anatomy and Physiology*, 15e. Chichester: Wiley.

Waugh, A. and Grant, A. (2018). *Ross and Wilson Anatomy and Physiology*. Edinburgh: Elsevier.

West, J.B. and Luks, A.M. (2015). *West's Respiratory Physiology*, 10e. Alphen aan den Rijn: Wolters Kluwer.

11

Research and evidence-based practice – 2

Contents

The first section on research and evidenced-based practice looked to give you a basic toolkit to help you in reading papers. Understanding the terms used in research can be complicated but becomes easier with the more you do it. This section will look to build on what you already know and look a little bit more in-depth at a few key topics within research.

Quantitative and qualitative

Quantitative research

- Provides numerical data for statistical analysis
- Typically for confirmatory studies
- Should be easily replicable
- Use tools and methods to generate numerical data
- Can be prospective or retrospective
- Do not usually allow for human interface with the research
- Statistics must be interpreted carefully in order to understand the research properly

Quantitative research

- Allows the researcher to explore the human interface
- Useful in exploratory studies

The Paramedic Revision Guide, First Edition. David W. Thom.
© 2021 John Wiley & Sons Ltd. Published 2021 by John Wiley & Sons Ltd.

- Typically prospective
- Can ask for written statements or gain information through face-to-face sessions
- Sessions may be structured, semi-structured or open
  - Structured enables the researcher to replicate exactly the interviews with each participant without deviation but does not allow the researcher or subject to explore the ideas within the study
  - Semi-structured may result in a less replicable interview but allows the subject to explore themes and ideas within and may provide insight
  - Open interviews may illicit a wide array of ideas and themes however may not be replicable
- Utilises thematic analysis
  - Can be manual or computer-generated
  - Identifies commonalities between answers given by the participants
  - Common ideas will be synthesised into a theme
  - That is, time pressures, lack of exposure, etc
- These themes can then often go on to inform further research or generate questions to be solved by quantitative research
- Qualitative research is complex to get right
  - Leading questions can skew results
  - Transcription errors may occur
  - Single participant versus groups can influence the level of detail and willingness to share
  - Choice of the interviewer may skew the participant's willingness to respond openly

> A common misconception is that one type of research is better than the other. In fact, both methods have their role in healthcare research.

Mixed methods

- Research may include both methods within the same study
- For example
  - A study may be looking at treatment options A versus treatment option B
  - Treatment B might statistically be the better option
  - However, the patients who received treatment B may report that they are more upset by or impacted by the treatment than those with option A
  - This may mean, depending on the significance of the benefit, that option B is not the right option going forwards.

Research terms

This section will look to add some more terms on top of what was covered in the first section (Table 11.1).

Randomisation

Randomisation is an area of research, whereby there is the possibility to introduce bias to research if not done carefully and correctly.

Randomisation is useful for also generating a wide spread of data amongst the participants as it will allow for the known and unknown variables within the participants.

Without randomisation, there is the potential for selection bias whereby the researcher could specifically pick participants for each group in order to generate the results desired.

Randomisation should be coupled with blinding so that the researcher or at the very least those interpreting the data are unable to determine facts on an individual participant.

Table 11.1 Research terms.

Research term	Explanation	Example
Homogeneity	Group of patients who have the same or similar traits or a similar variance that is useful to the research question	Patients of a similar age or who live in a specific location or have certain genetic variances that are specific to the research question and shared between all participants
Heterogeneity	Variance within the data set as a result of a diverse cohort. This may be clinical or methodological if looking at a review article.	Clinical variance may result in heterogeneity if the cohort includes a wide range of patients for example from differing genders, wide age range, differing socioeconomic status, epidemiological or genetic variance. Methodological heterogeneity may occur as a result of including multiple studies in a systematic review whereby the methods used to test a hypothesis may differ from each other or include a significant variation;
Null hypothesis	No difference can be detected and any difference is due to chance	Treatment A does not work. Any results that imply the treatment does work are down to chance
Alternative hypothesis	Contrary to a null hypothesis whereby difference is detected and not due to chance	Treatment B does work. Results that show this are not down to chance.
Type 1 error	False-positive result	Incorrect rejection of the null hypothesis. That is, believing that treatment A does work despite no evidence
Type 2 error	False-negative result	Incorrect acceptance of the null hypothesis. That is, believing Treatment B does not work despite evidence suggesting it does
Random error	Error introduced during the data collection	This could be down to poor procedures or individual variation in collection. This can be minimised by rigid protocols.
Sensitivity	Ability for a test to identify a disease	A highly sensitive test is likely to be positive if the disease is present and negative if it is not. Therefore, if the test is positive, there is a high probability of the patient having the disease
Specificity	Ability to identify those without a disease	A highly specific test is likely to be negative if the disease is not present. If a test is not specific it may produce a positive result caused by a different disease that is not the intended test. An example of this is the D-Dimer test that is highly sensitive for thromboembolic process but can also be raised in multiple other non-thromboembolic conditions therefore is not very specific.

Although there are multiple ways to randomise, there are a few commonly used methods, these are:

- Simple
- Block
- Stratified

Simple randomisation

- Usually, utilise computer-generated lists to assign participants a random number and then assign a treatment option to that number
- Do not follow any set pattern
- The most commonly used method for randomisation
- Can create unequal groups especially in smaller studies

Block

- Will allocate patients to a treatment option in blocks based upon their enrolment into the trial
    - That is, participants 1–10 are given treatment A, participants 11–20 are given treatment B, participants 21–30 are given treatment A, and so forth.
    - Block size can vary for each study but should remain constant during the study
- Allows for equal distribution into each study group
- If the researcher or patients determine the block size they may be able to surreptitiously chose their preferred treatment option

Stratified

- Less commonly used
- Typically utilised for smaller sample studies
- Allows for the patients or populations with pre-existing confounding factors to be equally distributed between groups

There are situations whereby normal randomisation methods are not suitable. This is particularly apparent in the ambulance service where multiple variables can affect the study before a patient is even reached. The 'PARAMEDIC' trial looking at the efficacy of the LUCAS® device found that they were unable to randomise through normal methods and adapted for continuing research in the ambulance service. More can be found in the reading list.

Sampling

As with randomisation, there are multiple methods of sampling that can be employed in healthcare research. Sampling is another area, whereby there is the possibility to introduce bias if not done correctly.

To determine the amount of participants required for the study a sample size calculation is performed, this will be informed by the size of the difference the researchers are looking to achieve as well as the prevalence of the disease or treatment within the population. The sample size is also affected by the power calculation.

The power of a study relates to how certain we can be that the results are not down to chance. This is typically set at a P value of 0.05 or a 5% chance the results are down to chance but a 95% chance they are not. If the researchers want to increase the certainty to a $P = 0.01$ or 1% chance this will take a greater sample size. These factors should be evident in the research study you are reading.

With sampling, there are a few quick points to remember

- If the difference is difficult to detect you will require more participants
- Small studies can only detect large differences
- Smaller studies are more likely to be affected by variations from the research protocol
- If a sample size/power calculation has been performed to ensure that the same number of patients are included in the statistical analysis
    - If the study has less patients calculated the study may be underpowered
    - An underpowered study may give false-positive or false-negative results
    - Studies may be stopped early due to clinical effect

Quick Questions

1. What is Heterogeneity?
2. Explain simple randomisation.
3. What is a type 2 error?

References and Further Reading

Abdull Wahab, S.F., Ismail, A.R., and Othman, R. (2018). Qualitative, quantitative or mixed: which is the most preferred for healthcare studies. In: *Advances in Human Factors and Ergonomics in Healthcare and Medical Devices*, vol. **590** (eds. V. Duffy and N. Lightner) (2017). Cham: Springer.

Allen, M. (2017). The SAGE encyclopedia of communication research methods. http://methods.sagepub.com/Reference/the-sage-encyclopedia-of-communication-research-methods (accessed 14 August 2020).

Galvin, I. (2018). Power and sample size. TBL. https://www.thebottomline.org.uk/blog/editorial/power-and-sample-size/ (accessed 15 August 2020).

Gates, S., Lall, R., Quinn, T. et al. (2017). Prehospital randomised assessment of a mechanical compression device in out-of-hospital cardiac arrest (PARAMEDIC): a pragmatic, cluster randomised trial and economic evaluation. *Health Technology Assessment* **21** (11): 1–176.

Goldacre, B. (2008). *Bad Science*. London: Fourth Estate.

Goldacre, B. (2013). *Bad Pharma*. London: Fourth Estate.

Higgins, J. and Thomas, J. (2019). *Cochrane Handbook for Systematic Reviews of Interventions*. Cochrane Training. https://training.cochrane.org/handbook/current (accessed 14 August 2020).

Mathieu, S. (2017). Type 1 and 2 errors. TBL. https://www.thebottomline.org.uk/blog/ebm/type-1-and-2-errors/ (accessed 14 August 2020).

Nickson, C. (2019a). Error in research. LITFL. https://litfl.com/error-in-research/ (accessed 14 August 2020).

Nickson, C. (2019b). Randomisation. LITFL. https://litfl.com/randomisation/ (accessed 15 August 2020).

Nickson, C. (2020). Statistical terms. LITFL. http://www.partone.litfl.com/statistical_terms.html (accessed 14 August 2020).

Perkins, G.D., Lall, R., Quinn, T. et al. (2015). Mechanical versus manual chest compression for out-of-hospital cardiac arrest (PARAMEDIC): a pragmatic, cluster randomised controlled trial. *The Lancet* **385**: 947–955.

West, S.L., Gartlehner G., Mansfield A.J. et al. (2010). Comparative effectiveness review methods: clinical heterogeneity. Agency for Healthcare Research and Quality. https://www.ncbi.nlm.nih.gov/books/NBK53310/ (accessed 14 August 2020).

Contents

This section will explore the factors affecting the decision-making as a paramedic as well as looking more in-depth at assessment. Although some of this will be a theoretical basis and may not seem overtly relevant, it should provide you with a basis for some of the subconscious processes that occur in practice.

It will build on techniques covered in 'Practical skills for Paramedics – 2' but may not repeat so it might be worth re-visiting the section if required. Some of the techniques may not be suitable for every patient but may be useful when dealing with patients with subtle or complex medical needs.

Decision theory

When making a diagnosis a number of factors may play into your thinking that may occur subconsciously. This forms the basis of diagnostic reasoning and decision theory. There are a number of models and theories that are proposed to identify traits within clinicians and assist in their processing of information.

Type 1 and Type 2 thinking

Type 1 thinking

- Fast
- Intuitive

The Paramedic Revision Guide, First Edition. David W. Thom.
© 2021 John Wiley & Sons Ltd. Published 2021 by John Wiley & Sons Ltd.

- Subconscious
- Automatic
- Pattern recognition
- Instinctive
- Emotional
- Based on previous experience
- Open to bias
- Act upon only the readily available information

Type 2 thinking

- Slow
- Thoughtful
- Considered
- Conscious process
- Logical
- Inquisitive
- Questioning
- Actively seeks more information than what is readily available

Cognitive pause

- Active process whereby the decision-maker forces a stop to their Type 1 thinking to allow time for Type 2
- Empowers the decision-maker and those around to question the initial decisions
- Cognizant 'sense check' on what the decision-maker is doing
- Encourages the decision-maker to seek other opinions

Why is this important?

When working as a paramedic, there will be instances where you will be required to make a rapid decision regarding a patient and a treatment option in order to preserve life and limb, that is, patient with impending airway compromise. With experience, this will fall into a Type 1 process whereby a rapid diagnosis and treatment plan will be made. This will be based on a system of pattern recognition and will become instinctive. It is important to actively include a cognitive pause, when appropriate, to ensure you are not blindly continuing down a single path without considering any alternatives or seeking help. The cognitive pause will encourage you to apply a Type 2 thought process and consider the situation more analytically with an open mind as well as encouraging you to seek the opinions of others who may already be applying a type 2 process.

Human reliability analysis

- The risk of error increases with the increased risk of complications
- Includes errors arising from human technology interfaces
- Error at any stage of the process can lead to errors in the following steps
- Wrong data going in = wrong endpoint

Why is this important?

The process of gathering data for patient assessment is done through both the history taking and the physical assessment. If you were to incorrectly interpret a piece of information at any point, this may lead to ultimately lead to the wrong diagnosis or treatment plan. Being cognizant that errors can creep in will encourage you to question your thought process or seek help from others if the risk associated from treatment is high.

In short, missed examination or misinterpreted information results in a misdiagnosis.

Dempster Shafer theory

- Multiple diagnoses considered concurrently
- The probability of each diagnosis is weighted
- Factors in for non-tangible effects and past experiences
- Groups of diagnoses can be excluded by additional information such as observations
- Involves a Type 2 thought process
- With experience, the weightings of diagnoses will change

Why is this important?

As a clinician when you assess a patient you will form a range of differential diagnoses at once. The Dempster–Shafer theory explains how you can consider all these diagnoses concurrently but as more information is gained you can weight each diagnosis with a probability it is correct. This will lead you to what you believe to be the most correct diagnosis and therefore the correct treatment plan. Although you may not consider the model by name when you are working, it shows that multiple diagnoses can be considered at once.

Bayes theorem

- Probability-based assessments
- Uses a degree of diagnostic insight that is then shown to be correct or incorrect
- If the diagnosis is shown to be correct by testing this will reinforce the belief that it is the correct diagnosis
- May exclude other diagnoses too early

Why is this important?

It is important to be aware that without forming a list of differential diagnoses, it is possible to reinforce an incorrect diagnosis at the exclusion of any other diagnoses.

Diagnostic reasoning

Making a diagnosis is part of working as a paramedic but there are some steps that you will go through in order to reach your diagnosis.

Diagnostic elements

- Knowledge of the patient
- Knowledge of the condition

- Knowledge of the treatment
- Identifying normal findings
- Identifying abnormal findings
  - Relevant and irrelevant
- The appearance of the patient
- Anatomical presentation
- Creation of a differential diagnosis list
- Test the hypothesis to form a working diagnosis
- Regular reassessment to ensure a correct diagnosis

Factors affecting diagnosis

- Past experience
- Education
- Personal biases
- Immediate thought processing
- Not engaging a Type 2 thought process
- Lack of information
- Failure to collect pertinent information
  - History taking
  - Observations
- Media

Why is this important?

By understanding that each clinician is fallible, it should encourage you to seek out as much information as possible before making a diagnosis.

Maxims of diagnosis

- The true disease presents itself
- Common diseases occur commonly
- Uncommon diseases occur uncommonly
- Uncommon manifestations of common diseases are more common than common manifestations of uncommon diseases

Why is this important?

Common diseases will present in a wide array of ways that may not fit rigid protocols or textbook definitions but this does not mean it is any less common.

References and Further Reading

Chen, L., Zhou, X., Xiao, F. et al. (2017). Evidential analytic hierarchy process dependence assessment methodology in human reliability analysis. *Nuclear Engineering and Technology* **49** (1): 123–133.

Ciabattoni, A., Muino, D.P., Vetterlein, T. et al. (2013). Formal approaches to rule-based systems in medicine. *International Journal of Approximate Reasoning* **54** (1): 132–148.

Cutler, D.M. and Zeckhauser, R.J. (1998). Adverse selection in health insurance. In: *Frontiers in Health Policy Research*, vol. **1** (ed. A.M. Garber), 1–32. Massachusetts: Massachusetts Institute of Technology: National Bureau of Economic Research.

Gigerenzer, G. and Gaissmaier, W. (2011). Heuristic decision making. *Annual Review of Psychology* **62**: 451–482.

Henderson, M., Tierney, L., and Smetana, G. (2012). *The Patient History: Evidence Based Approach*. New York: McGraw Hill.

Jones, R. (2017). Think twice. *British Journal of General Practice* **67** (665): 539.

Kahneman, D. (2011). *Thinking, Fast and Slow*. New York: Farrar, Straus and Giroux.

Katz, D. (2001). *Clinical Epidemiology and Evidence Based Medicine. Fundamental Principles of Clinical Reasoning and Research*. London: Sage.

Medow, M.A. and Lucey, C.R. (2011). A qualitative approach to Bayes' theorem. *BMJ Evidence-Based Medicine* **16** (6): 163–167.

Sox, H., Higgins, M., and Owens, D. (2013). *Medical Decision Making*, 2e. Chichester: Wiley Blackwell.

Patient consultation

The patient consultation is 'the central act of medicine' and will form a large part of your assessment and ultimately your time with the patient in order to form a diagnosis. The majority of 'ruling in' and 'ruling out' of diagnoses will be done during the history taking before any physical examination is made. A physical examination should be guided by a list of potential differential diagnoses in order to form a working diagnosis and treatment plan.

Purpose of the consultation

- Define the reason for attendance or seeking help
- Consider other problems that may be concomitant or underlying
- Work with the patient to generate an appropriate course of action for each problem
- Achieve a shared mental model of the problems and treatment options with the patient
- Involve the patient in the management of their condition and where appropriate encourage them to take responsibility for their health
- Utilise time and resources appropriately
- Establish or maintain clinical professional relationships in order for the patient to have confidence in yours and their ability to achieve goals

Preparing for the consultation

When assessing patients there are some important points to remember.
  The environment

- Privacy
    - It may be difficult but all efforts should be made
- The comfort of self and patient
- Eye-level if appropriate
- Respectful of personal space
- Equipment available to you

The clinician

- Your demeanour
- Your appearance
- Posture
- Verbal and non-verbal communication
- Cleanliness
- Presentation

Note taking

- There is a need to accurately and contemporaneously record information
- Be aware of distraction by documentation and diverting attention
- May miss cues if not paying attention to patient

Adapting the style

Paediatrics

- Give the child time
- Allow the child to build trust
- Work at their level
- Pitch your questions appropriate to their age
- Listen to the parent but also the child
- Be inquisitive and questioning

Elderly

- Give them time to explain but keep the examination focussed
- Be aware or visual and/or hearing loss
- Be aware of early symptoms of conditions associated with aging
- Consider the social situation as well as the patient

Introduction

- Wash your hands or apply hand gel as available
- Introduce yourself, give your clinical grade and reassurance
  - For example, 'Hello, my name is Dave. I'm a Paramedic from the Ambulance Service and I'm here to help'.
  - A small greeting and reassurance will go a long way
- Gain the patient's name and how they would like to be addressed
  - Some patients might prefer a shortened name or others may prefer a title such as Mr. or Miss. [surname]
- Gain consent for your consultation and assessment
- Ensure the patient is comfortable in their setting
- Presenting complaint
  - What has to lead them to seek help

Structuring the consultation (PHOSPHATE/SOCRATES)

There are multiple mnemonics available these are just some examples to help you ensure you gain a full history during your questioning. This works within the medical model of assessment covered in Chapter 2.

P-	Problem		**S-**	Site
H-	History (medical)		**O-**	Onset
O-	Onset		**C-**	Character
S-	Symptoms (associated)		**R-**	Radiation
P-	Precipitating factors		**A-**	Alleviating factors
H-	History (symptoms)		**T-**	Timing

A-	Alleviating/aggravating factors	E-	Exacerbating factors
T-	Timing	S-	Severity
E-	Aetiology		

Taking a family history (JAMi THREADS)

Family history is important as it may identify if the patient is at a genetic predisposition for a medical problem that might assist in your diagnosis. Here is a mnemonic to help you remember some of the things to ask if there is a family history.

J-	Jaundice or liver problems
A-	Asthma or breathing problems
Mi-	Myocardial infarction or other cardiac history
T-	Thyroid or endocrine problems
H-	Hypertension
R-	Renal problems or rheumatoid arthritis
E-	Epilepsy or similar
A-	Anaemia or other blood disorders
D-	Diabetes
S-	Stroke or serious illness such as cancer

211

Asking about alcohol

Chronic alcohol abuse can be insidious and unrecognised but can lead to serious health issues. It is important, where appropriate, to ask about the patient's alcohol history. CAGE is a screening tool for alcohol risk (Table 12.1).

Table 12.1   The CAGE assessment tool.

C-	Cutting down	Have you ever considered cutting down on your drinking?	Yes = 1
A-	Annoyed	Have you been annoyed by people asking about your drinking?	Yes = 1
G-	Guilty	Have you ever felt guilty about your drinking or the amount you drink?	Yes = 1
E-	Eye opener	Have you ever felt the need to have a drink first thing in the morning?	Yes = 1

A score greater than 2 is considered clinically significant.

Pertinent information

- Allergies
  - Medicines
  - Medical devices
- Drug history
  - Prescribed
  - Over the counter

- Recreational
- Current or previous abuse
- Social history
  - Non-verbal clues
  - Consider the environment
  - Document findings that may be pertinent to discharge, that is, home adaptions

Patient's viewpoint (ICE)

It may be pertinent to ask the patient what they consider to be the underlying problem; this may create a shared mental model so that both patient and clinician are aware of one another's worries and viewpoints.

I-   Impression. What is the patient's impression of their condition? What do they think it is?

C-   Concern. What is the patient most concerned about their condition and how can you help with this?

E-   Expectation. What is the patient's expectation of the care they are about to receive? Are they expecting to go to the hospital or be referred elsewhere?

Patient assessment

Physical assessment should be guided by your history taking with systems assessed systematically to ensure that key findings are not missed.

This has been covered in Chapter 2, and there are some additions within this section.

When it's not clear

Sometimes an immediate diagnosis is not clear. Although this may be frustrating this should not subtract from the clinical care the patient receives.

If you are unable to define a diagnosis the patient should be treated for the physiology that is presenting to you. There is a mnemonic that may help build a list of potential differentials, VITAMINS ABCDE.

V-   Vascular

I-   Infection/inflammatory

T-   Trauma

A-   Autoimmune/allergy

M-   Metabolic/mechanical

I-   Iatrogenic/idiopathic

N-   Neoplastic

S-   Social

A-   Alcohol

B-   Behavioural

C-   Congenital/chromosomal

D-   Degenerative/drugs

E-   Endocrine

Quick Questions

1. What does SOCRATES stand for?
2. When might you utilise the ICE pneumonic?

References and Further Reading

Bickley, L.S. (2013). *Bates' Guide to Physical Examination and History Taking*, 11e. Philidelphia: Wolters Kluwer.

Deveugele, M. et al. (2004). Consultation in general practice: a standard operating procedure? *Patient Education and Counselling* **54** (2): 227–233.

Douglas, G., Nicol, F., and Robertson, C. (2013). *Macleod's Clinical Examination*, 13e. Edinburgh: Churchill Livingstone Elsevier.

Ewing, J.A. (1984). Detecting alcoholism. The CAGE questionnaire. *JAMA* **252** (14): 1905–1907.

Gregory, P. and Ward, A. (2010). *Sanders' Paramedic Textbook*. Edinburgh: Mosby Elsevier.

Mehay, R. (2012). *The Essential Handbook for GP Training and Education*. London: Radcliffe Publishing.

Oxford Medical Education (2016). History taking – overview. OME. www.oxfordmedicaleducation.com/history/medical-general/ (accessed 17 August 2020).

Pendleton, D. (1984). *The Consultation: An Approach to Learning and Teaching*. Oxford: Open University Press.

Pendleton, D. et al. (2003). *The New Consultation: Developing Doctor-Patient Communication*. Oxford: Oxford University Press.

Rushforth, H. (2009). *Assessment Made Incredibly Easy!* Philidelphia: Wolters Kluwer.

Tate, P. (2009). *The Doctor's Communication Handbook*, 6e. Oxford: Radcliffe Publishing.

Zabidi-Hussin, Z.A. (2016). Practical way of creating differential diagnoses through an expanded VITAMINSABCDEK mnemonic. *Advances in Medical Education and Practice* **7**: 247–248.

Ear, Nose and Throat (ENT) assessment

The ENT system is complex but there are a few basics of assessment that should help you to manage patients presenting with an ENT condition. This section will cover the basics of anatomy as well as some techniques to help assess.

Anatomy of the ear

External

- Consists of:
  - Cartilage
  - Perichondrium
  - Skin
- Structures
  - Pinna (ear lobe)
  - External Auditory canal
- Functions
  - Collect and direct sound waves towards the middle ear
  - Wax producing glands
  - Hair protects middle ear structures

Middle Ear

- Structures
  - Tympanic membrane (Eardrum)
    - Pearly opaque in appearance
    - Amplifies and transmits sound to small bones (Ossicles)
  - Ossicles
    - Malleus (First)
- Attached to the inner surface of the tympanic membrane
    - Incus (Middle)
    - Stapes (Third)
- Attached to the opal window
  - Oval window
    - Demarcates between middle and inner ear structures

It is possible to dislocate ossicles with the most common being the Incus.

Inner ear

- Structures
  - Cochlea
    - Sound wave interpreter and converter
  - Vestibule
    - Contains utricle and saccule
    - Involved with motion
  - Three semi-circular canals
    - Sense rotational movement
  - Auditory nerves
  - Eustachian tubes

The Facial nerve passes through the middle ear in front of the mastoid process.

Taking an ear history

In addition to a standard medical history, there are some specifics to help you with your assessment. This list is by no means exhaustive but a good basis to start from.

- Pain (Otalgia)
  - Where?
  - Any Radiation
  - Aggravating and Alleviating factors
- Previous operations and or 'syringing'
- Any use of cotton buds
- Recent injury
- Recent flights
- Swimming and/or diving
- Discharge (Otorrhea)
  - How long?
  - Worsening?
  - Scanty or copious?
  - Smelly?
  - Bloodstained?
  - Watery?

- Hearing loss?
  - Onset time
  - Partial or complete
  - Bi-lateral/unilateral
  - Family history
  - Injury or surgery
  - Exposure to loud noises
- Vertigo
- Tinnitus

Assessment of the ear

This may be limited within your trust as not all allow invasive ear assessment by paramedics. Always refer to local policy before attempting assessment.

External ear

- Inspect healthy ear first
- Inspect auricle and mastoid process
  - Behind the ear
  - Looking for anything untoward including lumps, bumps or skin changes as well as wounds and bruising
- Inspect all other external structures
- Inspect for
  - Size and shape when compared to other ear
  - Symmetry
  - Trauma
  - Extra cartilage tags
  - Skin lesions/nodules/neoplasm/melanoma
  - Discharge (otorrhea)
  - Scars
  - Tenderness

Middle Ear

- Inspect using the otoscope (if trained and within local policy)
  - Hold otoscope in the same hand as ear inspecting
    - That is, left ear = left hand
  - Hold like a pencil placing the little finger on the patient to prevent any damage if the patient moves expectantly
  - Head tilted slightly away
  - Grasp pinna and gently pull up, out and back
    - Straightens the external ear structures
    - May cause the patient to cough due to stimulation of the cutaneous branch of the vagus nerve
- Assess all landmarks
  - Note canal for any inflammation
  - Move gently towards the tympanic membrane identifying landmarks as you advance until visible with membrane if possible.
  - Lateral process of malleus
  - Umbo of malleus
  - Incus

- The long process of malleus
- Pars Tensa
- Pars Flaccida
- Cone of light
  a. 5 o'clock in the right ear
  b. 7 o'clock in the left ear
- Assess for conditions such as:
  - Cerumen (wax)
    - May block your view of the structure
  - Cholesteatoma
    - Requires specialist review
  - Otitis media
  - Effusion
  - Fluid behind the drum
  - Blocked Eustachian tube
  - Perforated membrane
  - Grommets (tympanostomy)

Basic hearing test

Hearing can be both conductive and sensorineural, the two should be tested if testing hearing. For most conditions you will encounter as a paramedic a simple 'can you hear me' would be sufficient but there are a few simple additional tests that can be performed to narrow the diagnosis

Whisper test (Conductive).

- Cover each ear in turn and whisper '123' and 'abc'
- Ask the patient what they heard

Rhomberg test (Sensorineural)

- Ask the patient to stand up, eyes closed, feet together
- Assess for swaying

Rinne test (Conductive)

- Bone conduction (BC) versus air conduction (AC)
- Air should be better than bone
- Tuning fork struck and then placed on mastoid process, struck again and placed by ear
  - Ask patient which is louder/clearer
- Rinne test positive (Normal hearing) when AC > BC
- Rinne test negative when BC > AC
  - Possible conductive hearing loss
- False negatives in presence of a 'non-hearing' ear

Webber test (Conductive/Sensorineural)

- Strike tuning fork
- Place tuning form on patient's central forehead or skull
- Sound will be heard in-ear presenting with reduced hearing

- Sound hear equally in both ears
    - Positive Webber
    - Normal hearing
- The sound heard in the affected ear
    - Possible unilateral conductive hearing loss due to middle ear pathology
- Sound hear in the unaffected ear
    - Unilateral Sensorineural hearing loss

Anatomy of the nose

External

- Structures
    - Root
    - Bridge
    - Dorsum nasi
    - Nasofacial angle
    - Apex (tip)
    - Naris (nostril)
    - Septum
    - Philtrum
    - Nasal sulcus
- Functions
    - Protection
    - Support

Internal

- Structures
    - Upper/middle/lower turbinate
    - Paranasal sinuses
    - Nasolacrimal duct drainage
    - Olfactory nerves in the roof
    - Kiesselbachs plexus/littles area in anterior nose of septum
        - The most common site for anterior epistaxis
    - Sphenopalatine artery branches behind middle turbinate
        - A common site for posterior epistaxis
- Functions
    - Warm and humidify air
    - Filter large particulates
    - Mucous production
    - Olfactory sense

Taking a nose history

- Duration of symptoms
- Aggravating/Alleviating symptoms
- Allergies/Atopic disease
- Smoking/Illicit drug use

- Any pets as home
- Occupation
- Previous surgery
- Trauma
- General medical history
- Seasonal/daily variation of symptoms
- Discharge
- Changes in sense of taste or smell

Assessment of the nose

Again, this may be limited within your trust, refer to local policy before attempting invasive assessment.

External

- Skin
  - Does it match the facial complexion?
  - Any coarseness or flaking
  - Any lesions
  - Redness
- Abnormal creases
- Shape/symmetry
- Nares/septum midline and symmetrical
- Palpate nasal bones
  - Tenderness
  - Deformity
- Palpate sinuses

Internal

- Inspect using the otoscope (if trained and within local policy)
- Be cautious as you advance not to cause trauma to the nose or pain
- Assess nasal landmarks
  - Nasal septum
  - Turbinate
    - Pink in appearance
    - Sensitive
    - Likely to only spot the inferior turbinate
- Assess for
  - Swelling
  - Lesions
  - Inflammation
  - Deformity
  - Discharge
  - Foreign bodies
  - Bleeding points or wounds
  - Haematomas
  - Erosion
  - Polyps

Anatomy of the mouth and throat

- Lips
- Gums
- Teeth
- Labial frenulum
- Tongue
- Frenulum linguae
- Hard palate
- Soft palate
- Uvula
- Tongue
- Tonsils

Taking a mouth and throat history

- Dry/cracking lips
- Sores/Ulcerations
- Swelling
- Noticed any thick white coating
- White plaques on the buccal mucosa
- Lesions or lumps on lips or mucosa
- Duration of pain/symptoms
- Severity
- Aggravating and alleviating factors
- Localised pain or diffuse
- Any other illness
- Medication including inhalers
- Smoking status
- Alcohol consumption
- Diet/weight loss
- Voice changes
- Swallowing difficulties
- Changes in taste

Assessment of the mouth and throat

This may vary by trust always refer to local policy. If there is a concern regarding epiglottitis there should not be any instrumentation of the airway. If there is the risk of actual or impending airway compromise, then this should be managed as a priority. Be aware of other conditions that may present with mouth and throat symptoms such as anaphylaxis.

Assess the mouth

- Lips
  - Lesions
  - Cracking
  - Abnormal pigmentation
- Labial Frenulum
  - Connects each lip to the gingiva
  - Observe colour, texture, swelling and abnormalities
  - Wounds or injury

- Dental structure
  - Oral hygiene
  - Decay
  - Gum inflammation
  - Breath
  - Bleeding
- Tongue
  - Colour/texture
  - Moist
  - Any abnormalities
- Buccal mucosa
  - Pink/moist
  - Any lacy white patches
- Inguinal frenulum
  - Attaches bottom of the tongue to the floor of the mouth
  - Intact
  - Lesions
- Any ulceration
- Thrush
- Test cranial nerve XII

Assess the throat

- Using a tongue depressor and a torch
- Inspect
  - Posterior pharynx
  - Tonsils
  - Uvula
  - All other visible structures
- Should appear moist and pink
- Say 'Ahh'
  - Assess for symmetry
  - Assesses cranial nerves IX and X
- Soft and hard palates intact?
- Tonsillitis
- Pharyngitis
- Abscesses

References and Further Reading

Bickley, L.S. (2013). *Bates' Guide to Physical Examination and History Taking*, 11e. Philidelphia: Wolters Kluwer.

Corbridge, R.J. (2011). *Essential ENT*, 2e. London: Hodder Arnold.

Douglas, G., Nicol, F., and Robertson, C. (2013). *Macleod's Clinical Examination*, 13e. Edinburgh: Churchill Livingstone Elsevier.

Gregory, P. and Ward, A. (2010). *Sanders' Paramedic Textbook*. Edinburgh: Mosby Elsevier.

Ludman, H.S. and Bradley, P.J. (2012). *ABC of Ear, Nose and Throat*. Chichester: Wiley Blackwell.

Peate, I. and Nair, M. (2016). *Fundamentals of Anatomy and Physiology: For Nursing and Healthcare Students*, 2e. Chichester: Wiley Blackwell.

Rushforth, H. (2009). *Assessment Made Incredibly Easy!* Philidelphia: Wolters Kluwer.

Sami, A.S. (2017). *ENT Made Easy*. Banbury: Scion Publishing.

Tortora, G.J. and Derrickson, B.H. (2017). *Tortora's Principles of Anatomy and Physiology*, 15e. Chichester: Wiley.

Waugh, A. and Grant, A. (2018). *Ross and Wilson Anatomy and Physiology*. Edinburgh: Elsevier.

Eye assessment

Injuries to the eye can arise from a range of situations including blunt force trauma, penetrating trauma, foreign objects, chemicals and contact lenses. This section is to give you the basics of an eye assessment but should not delay a patient from reaching definitive care. Sight loss due to an eye injury can have devastating impacts for a patient. Refer to local policy for local variation.

Basic anatomy

- Lids
- Tear ducts
- Sclera
- Iris
- Pupil
- Conjunctiva
- Cornea
- Anterior chamber

Eye history

- When did it happen?
- How did it happen
- Associated and non-associated ocular symptoms
- Past ocular history combined with medical/surgical history
- Family history
- Drug history
- Allergies
- Any action is taken prior to arrival
- First-aid measures
- Are spectacles or lenses worn normally?
- If so, were they have worn at the time of injury?
- If a chemical injury do, they have a sample of the substance
- Loss of vision
    - Sudden or gradual
    - Painful or painless
    - Transient or permanent
    - Bilateral or unilateral
    - Part or all of the visual field
- Red-eye
    - Watery or sticky
    - Painful or painless
    - Visual loss
    - Duration
- Photophobia

Assessment of the eye

Inspection

- Surrounding skin
- Lid swelling
    - Inflammation or haematoma

- Eye closing
- Dryness
- Oedema
- Lesion
- Lacerations
- Blood
- Debris
- Hyphema
  - Blood in the anterior chamber
- Iris
  - Central
  - Round
- Pupil

Visual acuity

- Snellen chart
  - May have to improvise pre-hospital
    - Using a newspaper at arm's length is a good improvisation working from the headline to the smallest text
  - If the patient normally wears glasses these should be worn
  - Each eye tested individually
  - If patients can't see the chart then hold fingers at 50 cm and ask if the patient is able to see them
  - If patients can't see fingers then wave a hand in front of the patient to assess if they can see movement
  - If unable to see movement test pupil reaction

Fields of Vision

- Test each eye separately
- Sit a comfortable distance from the patient-facing each other
- Ask the patient to look at the tip of your nose
- Using the tip of your finger work from the outermost point towards the nose equidistant from you and the patient
- Use your own vision as the benchmark if the normal field of vision
- Ask the patient to say yes when they can see your finger
- This should be repeated on each side and top/bottom of vision for both eyes independently

Eye function

- Pupil reaction
  - Direct and indirect
- H-gaze
- Near/far focus

References and Further Reading

Bickley, L.S. (2013). *Bates' Guide to Physical Examination and History Taking*, 11e. Philidelphia: Wolters Kluwer.

Douglas, G., Nicol, F., and Robertson, C. (2013). *Macleod's Clinical Examination*, 13e. Edinburgh: Churchill Livingstone Elsevier.

Gregory, P. and Ward, A. (2010). *Sanders' Paramedic Textbook*. Edinburgh: Mosby Elsevier.

Peate, I. and Nair, M. (2016). *Fundamentals of Anatomy and Physiology: For Nursing and Healthcare Students*, 2e. Chichester: Wiley Blackwell.

Rushforth, H. (2009). *Assessment Made Incredibly Easy!* Philidelphia: Wolters Kluwer.

Tortora, G.J. and Derrickson, B.H. (2017). *Tortora's Principles of Anatomy and Physiology*, 15e. Chichester: Wiley.

Waugh, A. and Grant, A. (2018). *Ross and Wilson Anatomy and Physiology*. Edinburgh: Elsevier.

Whittaker, J.D. (2017). Eye – initial assessment. https://www.rcemlearning.co.uk/reference/eye-initial-assessment/ (accessed 13 January 2021).

Respiratory assessment

This section will look to add a few additional skills to your respiratory assessment. This should be used in conjunction with the skills previously covered but might mean you are able to illicit more information through your assessment. Refer to local policy for regional variations.

Inspection

The inspection section of the assessment is not limited to the chest itself but taking a global view of the patient.

- Finger clubbing
  - Not specific to lung disease
- Palmar Erythema
  - Not specific to lung disease
- CO_2 retention 'flap'
  - It may be confused with liver flap in concurrent illness
- Breathlessness
- Additional pillows at night/sleeping in a chair?
- Chest shape
  - Anterior-Posterior distance increased in chronic hyperinflation lung disease
- Scars
- Masses
- Cyanosis

Palpation

- Lung excursion
- Chest expansion front and back
- Equal rise and fall?
- Lymph nodes

Tactile vocal fremitus

- Gain consent
- Chaperone
- Expose as appropriate
- The patient sat upright with arms folded across chest
- Place palms lightly on the patients back with your fingers splayed away so the only palm in contact
  - Utilise the ulnar borders of both hands (sides of hand) if this is uncomfortable
- Ask the patient to repeat the phrase 'ninety-nine' loud enough that vibrations can be felt in the chest wall
- Repeat in all areas of the lungs mindful of patient dignity and avoiding personal areas

- Vibrations should feel equal on each side
  - More intense vibrations may indicate consolidation at that site
  - Less intense vibrations may indicate air-filled lung such as emphysema or pneumothorax

Auscultation

Vocal fremitus

- Can be assessed if adventitious (added) sounds have been identified on initial auscultation
- Listening for vocal sounds and abnormal transmission of voice if consolidation is present

Bronchophony

- The patient repeats the phrase 'Ninety Nine' whilst auscultating all fields
- In normal lung tissue, the sound will appear muffled
- Consolidation will cause words to sound abnormally loud

Egophony

- Ask the patient to say, and maintain, sound 'eeeeeeee…' whilst auscultating all fields
- In normal lung tissue, the sound will be muffled
- Consolidation will cause it to sound like 'aaaaaaaa…'

Whispered pectoriloquy

- Ask the patient to repeatedly whisper the phrase '1, 2, 3' whilst auscultating all fields
- In normal lung tissue, the sound will be almost inaudible
- Consolidation will cause it to sound loud and clear

References and Further Reading

Bickley, L.S. (2013). *Bates' Guide to Physical Examination and History Taking*, 11e. Philidelphia: Wolters Kluwer.

Douglas, G., Nicol, F., and Robertson, C. (2013). *Macleod's Clinical Examination*, 13e. Edinburgh: Churchill Livingstone Elsevier.

Gregory, P. and Ward, A. (2010). *Sanders' Paramedic Textbook*. Edinburgh: Mosby Elsevier.

Newnham, M., Jones, E., Wall, D., and Mukherjee, R. (2011). The reliability of the respiratory physical examination. *Thorax* **66** (supplement): A143.

Peate, I. and Nair, M. (2016). *Fundamentals of Anatomy and Physiology: For Nursing and Healthcare Students*, 2e. Chichester: Wiley Blackwell.

Rushforth, H. (2009). *Assessment Made Incredibly Easy!* Philidelphia: Wolters Kluwer.

Seidel, H.M., Ball, J.W., Flynn, J.A. et al. (2010). *Mosby's Guide to Physical Examination*, 7e. Missouri: Elsevier.

Serrao, R., Zirwas, M., and English, J.C. (2007). Palmar erythema. *American Journal of Dermatology* **8** (6): 347–356.

Tortora, G.J. and Derrickson, B.H. (2017). *Tortora's Principles of Anatomy and Physiology*, 15e. Chichester: Wiley.

Waugh, A. and Grant, A. (2018). *Ross and Wilson Anatomy and Physiology*. Edinburgh: Elsevier.

Wong, C.L., Holroyd-Leduc, J., and Straus, S.E. (2009). Does this patient have pleural effusion? *Journal of the American Medical Association* **301** (3): 309–317.

Cardiovascular assessment

This section will look to add a few additional skills to your cardiovascular assessment. This should be used in conjunction with the skills previously covered but might mean you are able to illicit more information through your assessment. Refer to local policy for regional variations.

Inspection

- Clubbing
  - Not specific to cardiovascular disease
- Splinter haemorrhages
  - Indicative of endocarditis
- Osler's nodes
  - Small tender swellings in fingertips
  - Indicative of endocarditis
- Janeway lesions
  - Septic emboli cause micro-abscesses seen on palms
  - May also seen on soles of feet
- Evidence of Marfan's syndrome?
- Ross spots
  - Haemorrhagic spots to the conjunctiva
  - Indicative of endocarditis
- Xanthelasma
  - White plaque-like build-up
  - Indicative of hypercholesterolaemia
- Corneal arcus
  - White rings around the iris
  - Indicative of hypercholesterolaemia
- Frank sign
  - Deep grove within the ear lobe
  - Indicative of high cholesterol

Jugular venous pressure

- Use the right internal jugular vein (IJV)
- The patient should be sat at 45°
- IJV should not be visible when standing
- Ask the patient to turn their head slightly to the left
- Locate surface markings of the IJV
  - Runs from the medial end of the clavicle to the ear lobe under the medial aspect of sternomastoid muscles
- If visible
- Look for a double waveform pulsation
- Waveform will be visible but not palpable
- May help to palpate the contralateral carotid pulse to differentiate
- Measure the level of the JVP by measuring the vertical distance between the sternal angle and the top of where the pulsating JVP is visible
- Normally 4–5 cm

Palpation

Palpate for the Apex

- Apex is the palpable pulsation of the heart
- Assess for the furthest outwards and the downwards point where this is felt
- Normally found between the 6th and 8th intercostal space mid-clavicular
- Moves with patient positioning for 45° semi-recumbent is best

- Forceful apex?
  - Increased cardiac output
  - Possible sepsis or exercise-induced
- Diffuse apex?
  - Poor left ventricle function
  - Possible congestive cardiac failure

Palpating for Thrills

- Palpate over where valves should anatomically be
- Assess for a palpable murmur
- May feel like a vibration or a 'purring'

Auscultation

It may be possible to hear additional sounds or murmurs on auscultation although their diagnosis may be complex and require further investigations. As a rule, a patient with a new or undiagnosed murmur should be admitted to the hospital for further investigation as some may have severe consequences if left untreated or may be a sign of underlying acute or chronic pathology.

Murmurs may be

- Continuous
- Mid-systolic
- Pan-systolic
- Early diastolic
- Mid-diastolic
- Pre-systolic

Further information on heart murmurs can be found in the reading list.

References and Further Reading

Bickley, L.S. (2013). *Bates' Guide to Physical Examination and History Taking*, 11e. Philidelphia: Wolters Kluwer.

Douglas, G., Nicol, F., and Robertson, C. (2013). *Macleod's Clinical Examination*, 13e. Edinburgh: Churchill Livingstone Elsevier.

Farkas, J. (2016). The Internet book of critical care. EMCrit. https://emcrit.org/ibcc/toc/ (accessed 21 August 2020).

Gregory, P. and Ward, A. (2010). *Sanders' Paramedic Textbook*. Edinburgh: Mosby Elsevier.

Nickson, C. (2019). Murmurs DDx. LITFL. https://litfl.com/murmurs-ddx/ (accessed 21 August 2020).

Peate, I. and Nair, M. (2016). *Fundamentals of Anatomy and Physiology: For Nursing and Healthcare Students*, 2e. Chichester: Wiley Blackwell.

Rushforth, H. (2009). *Assessment Made Incredibly Easy!* Philidelphia: Wolters Kluwer.

Seidel, H.M., Ball, J.W., Flynn, J.A. et al. (2010). *Mosby's Guide to Physical Examination*, 7e. Missouri: Elsevier.

Tortora, G.J. and Derrickson, B.H. (2017). *Tortora's Principles of Anatomy and Physiology*, 15e. Chichester: Wiley.

Waugh, A. and Grant, A. (2018). *Ross and Wilson Anatomy and Physiology*. Edinburgh: Elsevier.

Musculoskeletal assessment

This section will provide a basis for some of the basics of musculoskeletal assessment.

Extra anatomical terms

Circumduction

- Move joint in 360°
  - That is, rotation of the wrist

Circumferential

- Surrounds in a ring

Pronation

- Turn palm down

Supination

- Turn palm up

Palmar/Volvar surface

- The surface that is visible on the arms when the palms are facing forwards

Dorsal/extensive surface

- Everything behind the palmar surface

Ulnar deviation

- Where the wrist, kept flat, is bent towards the little finder side

Radial deviation

- Where the wrist is bent towards to thumb side

Generic joint examination

Look, Feel, Move.

1. Look
   a. Skin colour
   b. Scars
   c. Rashes
   d. Swelling
   e. Muscle Wasting
   f. Deformity

2. Feel
   a. Skin temp
   b. Swelling (hard/soft/fluctuant)
   c. Tenderness
3. Move
   a. Active/passive/restricted movements
   b. Abnormal movements
4. Other stability tests

Shoulder assessment

Rotator cuff muscles

- Supraspinatus – Abduction
- Infrascapularis – External rotation
- Teres Minor – External rotation
- Subscapularis – Internal rotation

> **S.I.T.S.**
> Useful acronym for remembering the muscles of the rotator cuff.

Consider causes of pain

- Rotator cuff
- Instability
- Acromion-Clavicular Joint (AC Joint)
- Referred pain

Common causes of pain

- Rotator cuff strain
- Tendinopathy
- Glenohumeral dislocation
- Glenohumeral instability
- Tears
- C-spine
- T-spine
- Soft tissue injury
- AC Joint sprain

History taking

- SOCRATES
- Any pain at night
- Previous treatment
- Family history
- Systemic symptoms

Examination

- Look
  - Deformity
  - Asymmetry

228

- Wasting
- Bruising
- Scars
  - Tip of the shoulder for a possible supraspinatus tear
  - Multiple keyholes for AC Joint repair
- Feel
  - Start at sterno-clavicular joint
  - Feel along clavicle to AC joint
  - Around acromion to head of humerus
  - Feel around the back from AC joint to the scapula
    - Scapula fractures carry a high risk of serious thoracic injury
  - Feel long head of biceps
    - Local tenderness of bicipital grove
  - Greater tuberosity
    - Local tenderness increases the probability of fracture
  - Spine of scapula
    - Local tenderness increases the probability of fracture
- Move
  - Range of movement
    - Flexion
    - Extension
    - Adduction
    - Abduction
  - Limited active but full passive?
    - Possible rotator cuff tear or supraspinatus impingement
  - Limited active and passive
    - Possible adhesive capsulitis
  - Painful abduction worsening at 60°+
    - Supraspinatus impingement/rotator cuff

Examining the Supraspinatus

- Abduction and internal/external rotation
  - Stand patient up with arms by their side
  - Stand behind the patient
  - Flex elbow to 90°
  - Locate Acromion and place your fingers anteriorly to this
  - Bring arm back
    - Will be painful if inflamed
    - Relieved by bringing arm forwards
  - Bring patients arms out to their side and rotate thumbs downwards
  - Push down on arms
    - Assess for weakness
  - Abduct arm through a full range
    - 60°–90° will be pain-free
    - 90°–120° painful then becomes pain-free again
    - Confirms diagnosis

Supraspinatus strength

- The patient put arms out in front and apart
- Turn thumbs inwards
- Removes the power of the pectoral chest muscles
- Rest your hands on theirs
- Ask the patient to push against your hands
- Patients with Supraspinatus damage will show with deficit to one side

Infraspinatus/Teres Minor

- Arms by the patient's side elbows flexed to 90°
- Place your hands on the patients' elbows
- Ask the patient to push out against hands
  - Painful
  - Assess for unilateral deficit

Subscapularis (Internal rotators)

- Ask the patient to put their hand behind their back
  - Removes the power of the pectoral muscles
- Put the back of their hand on their back
- Place your palm on theirs
- Ask them to push against your palm
- Do both sides and assess for deficit?

Scapula 'winging'

- Can be normal in children
- Ask the patient to do a 'press up' whilst standing against a wall
- Observe to see if the scapula moves away from the chest wall
- Suggests nerve damage to the rhomboids and serratus anterior

Examining the elbow

Look

- Swelling
- Colour
- Scars
- Compare to the other arm
- Olecranon bursae
  - Observe for undue swelling

Feel

- Swelling
- Ask the patient to flex the elbow
  - Feel for an isosceles triangle

- Ask the patient to extend the elbow
  - Triangle should be in one line

Move

- Extension and flexion
- Supinate and Pronate

The ottawa knee rules

The Ottawa knee rules are a series of examination and clinical decision tools that aids in the determination of the need for medical imaging (X-Ray) following trauma. They are primarily used for acute trauma within the last seven days and are less sensitive to chronic pathology.

X-Ray is indicated only if there is an injury with any of the following:

- Age greater than 55
  (OR)
- Isolated tenderness of the patella and no other structures
  (OR)
- Tenderness of the head of the fibula
  (OR)
- Cannot flex to 90°
  (OR)
- Unable to weight bear immediately or for four steps during the assessment

Patella tenderness is only significant if isolated

Limping counts as bearing weight as long as weight is transferred twice onto each lower limb (four steps).

The ottawa ankle rules

The Ottawa ankle rules determine the need for medical imaging following ankle or foot trauma. Although the foot and ankle are imaged separately, the rules may be considered together in your assessment.

X-Ray is indicated only if there is an injury with any of the following:

Ankle

- Bony tenderness over the lateral malleolus
  (OR)
- Bony tenderness over the medial malleolus
  (OR)
- Inability to weight bear immediately or more than four steps during an assessment

Foot

- Bony tenderness at the base of the 5th metatarsal
  (OR)
- Bony tenderness over the navicular
  (OR)
- Inability to weight bear immediately or more than four steps during the assessment

231

Clinical judgment should supersede the rules if the patient:

- Is intoxicated or uncooperative
- Has other distracting painful injuries
- Has diminished sensation in their legs
- Has gross swelling which prevents palpation of the malleolar bone tenderness

Note:

- During the assessment you should also palpate the fibula and tibia
- Medial malleolus tenderness should not be ignored
- Limping counts as weight-bearing
- Be cautious in applying the rules to patients under age 18

Hand examination
Useful terminology
   Hand

- Supination = Palm up
- Pronation = Palm down

Fingers

- Flexion = curl inwards
- Extension = straighten
- Hyperextension = bend backwards
- Abduction = fan-out
- Adduction = close in

Thumb

- Extension = straighten 'thumbs-up'
- Flexion = curl inwards
- Opposition = touch thumb to the little finger
- Palmar abduction = palm up and lift thumb up
- Radial abduction = thumbs up away from the radius

Wrist

- Extension = bend back
- Flexion = bend inwards
- Ulnar deviation = hand on flat plane bend outwards
- Radial deviation = hand on flat plane bend inwards

Assessment

- Ask
  - SOCRATES
  - Dominant hand
  - Occupation
  - Remove jewellery if able
- Look
  - Top of hand
    - Scars
    - Deformities
    - Nodes
    - Skin
    - Muscles
    - Nails
  - Palms
    - Scars
    - Muscle wasting
    - Palmar erythema
    - Swellings
  - Forearm
    - Muscle bellies for hand muscles are found in the forearm
    - Swellings
    - Lumps
    - Scars
  - General hand health
    - Any obvious deformities or deviations
- Feel
  - Ask about pain
  - Palms
  - Top of hand
  - Warmth
  - Any specific heat points over joints
  - Palpate all joints and tendons
- Move (active/passive/resisted)
  - Assess for the limited range of movement as well as pain and crepitus
  - Wrist
    - Flexion/extension
    - Pronation/supination
    - Deviation
  - Fingers
    - Flexion/extension
    - Splay fingers out
  - Thumb
    - Flexion/extension
    - Opposition
    - Abduction

- Sensation
  - Assess sharp/dull sensation in all plains and nerve distribution
- Power
  - Check strength in all plains of movement
- Special tests
  - Phalen's test
    - Reverse Prayer sign for one minute
    - Positive if causes pain/paraesthesia
  - Tap the median nerve pathway in the wrist
    - Positive if causes paraesthesia

Heberden's nodes

- Swelling/Nodes on distal interphalangeal joint
- Associated with osteoarthritis

Bouchard's nodes

- Swelling/Nodes on proximal interphalangeal joint
- Associated with osteoarthritis
- Found in rheumatoid arthritis

References and Further Reading

Bickley, L.S. (2013). *Bates' Guide to Physical Examination and History Taking*, 11e. Philidelphia: Wolters Kluwer.

Douglas, G., Nicol, F., and Robertson, C. (2013). *Macleod's Clinical Examination*, 13e. Edinburgh: Churchill Livingstone Elsevier.

Gregory, P. and Ward, A. (2010). *Sanders' Paramedic Textbook*. Edinburgh: Mosby Elsevier.

Mansbridge, C. (2013). Orthopaedic/hematological hand and wrist examination. OSCEstop. https://oscestop.com/Hand_exam.pdf (accessed 21 August 2020).

Peate, I. and Nair, M. (2016). *Fundamentals of Anatomy and Physiology: For Nursing and Healthcare Students*, 2e. Chichester: Wiley Blackwell.

Rushforth, H. (2009). *Assessment Made Incredibly Easy!* Philidelphia: Wolters Kluwer.

Seidel, H.M., Ball, J.W., Flynn, J.A. et al. (2010). *Mosby's Guide to Physical Examination*, 7e. Missouri: Elsevier.

Stiell, I.G. et al. (1994). Implementation of the Ottawa ankle rules. *JAMA* **271**: 827–832.

Stiell, I.G. et al. (1995). A multicentre trial to introduce clinical decision rules for the use of radiography in acute ankle injuries. *British Medical Journal* **311**: 594–597.

Stiell, I.G., Wells, G.A., Hoag, R.H. et al. (1997). Implementation of the Ottawa knee rule for the use of radiography in acute knee injuries. *JAMA* **278** (23): 2075–2079.

Tortora, G.J. and Derrickson, B.H. (2017). *Tortora's Principles of Anatomy and Physiology*, 15e. Chichester: Wiley.

Waugh, A. and Grant, A. (2018). *Ross and Wilson Anatomy and Physiology*. Edinburgh: Elsevier.

234

13

Pre-hospital trauma

Contents

Whilst major trauma is relatively uncommon in UK civilian practice, lesser trauma is a regular occurrence. Trauma should be considered as both a physical and mental injury and can occur from a wide array of circumstances. At each end of the age spectrum, the response to trauma varies greatly, and it takes a lesser mechanism to result in life-threatening injuries. This section will look at some of the basics of trauma management. A 'trauma survey' has been covered in 'Practical Skills for Paramedics – 2', and this section will look to build upon this.

Physics in trauma

Although as a paramedic physics may not immediately spring to mind when considering trauma but there are a few basic principles that are pertinent to trauma. These are kinetic energy and the transfer of energy.

Kinetic energy

Kinetic energy describes the forces that act upon a moving object. It is demonstrated as follows:

$$KE = \frac{1}{2}mv^2,$$

Whereby 　KE - Kinetic Energy
　　　　　m - Mass in kilograms
　　　　　v - Velocity in meters per second

Kinetic energy is described in the unit kilogram meter squared per second squared or 'kgm^2/s^2'
　　So why is this applicable?

The Paramedic Revision Guide, First Edition. David W. Thom.
© 2021 John Wiley & Sons Ltd. Published 2021 by John Wiley & Sons Ltd.

Well, consider an average 70 kg cyclist on a road traveling at 20 km/hr falling off. Their kinetic energy before the impact is as follows:

$$\frac{1}{2} \times 70\,kg \times 5.6^2\,m/s \quad (20\,km/hr \text{ is approx. } 5.6\,m/s)$$

Which is the same as as follows:

$$\frac{1}{2} \times 70\,kg \times 31.36\,m/s = 1097.6\,kgm^2/s^2$$

However, if the speed of the cyclist is increased slightly to 30 km/hr:

$$\frac{1}{2} \times 70\,kg \times 8.4^2\,m/s \quad (30\,km/hr \text{ is approx. } 8.4\,m/s)$$

Which is the same as follows:

$$\frac{1}{2} \times 70\,kg \times 70.56\,m/s = 2469.6\,kgm^2/s^2$$

By increasing the speed by just 10 km/hr the kinetic energy is over doubled which will result in a greater force applied to the patient on impact.

To use a different example, consider a patient walking at a normal pace into a stationary lorry. For argument, we use a standard 7.5-ton lorry as commonly seen in the UK.

$$\frac{1}{2} \times 70\,kg \times 1.4^2\,m/s \quad (5\,km/hr \text{ is approx. } 1.4\,m/s)$$

Which is the same as follows:

$$\frac{1}{2} \times 70\,kg \times 1.96\,m/s = 68.6\,kgm^2/s^2$$

However, if we now make the person stationary and the lorry traveling at the walking pace the equation looks like this:

$$\frac{1}{2} \times 7500\,kg \times 1.4^2\,m/s$$

Which is the same as follows:

$$\frac{1}{2} \times 7500\,kg \times 1.96\,m/s = 7350\,kgm^2/s^2$$

By changing the moving part but keeping the other factors, the same the kinetic energy involved is now vastly greater than previous.

To extend the analogy further lets consider the same pedestrian being hit by the same lorry at a speed of just 12 mph (approx. 20 km/hr) such as a lorry driving slowly along city streets.

$$\frac{1}{2} \times 7500\,kg \times 5.6^2\,m/s \quad (20\,km/hr \text{ is approx } .5.6\,m/s)$$

Which is the same as follows:

$$\frac{1}{2} \times 7500\,\text{kg} \times 31.36\,\text{m/s} = 117600\,\text{kgm}^2/\text{s}^2$$

This demonstrates that even at low speeds there can be tremendous energy generated that could be transferred to the patient. With increased energy comes an increase in the chance of serious injury or death. Compare the same speed for cycling and the lorry.

Now I know these equations are crude and there will be some with a far greater knowledge of physics than me who will, rightly, point out that these do not allow for additional factors such as the impact vectors and trajectories but the basic principles are enough for what we are trying to achieve. With increased mass and/or speed the kinetic energy and therefore energy transferred will be increased. After all, we are Paramedics not Physicists.

Transfer of energy

For the energy to cause injury, it must be transferred into the patient. Once the energy has been transferred to the patient, it can be transferred between the tissues of the body causing further injury.
Two examples of energy transfer are vehicle collisions and fall from height onto the feet.

Vehicle collisions

- Whilst traveling in the car there is potential energy within the person which will remain constant until acted upon
- If the vehicle impacts a solid object, that is oncoming vehicle or another structure it sustains a rapid deceleration, the potential energy is converted to kinetic energy resulting in the movement of the person within the vehicle
- If the person then is restrained by the seatbelt or impacts with the inside of the car, the energy is then transferred to the internal organs resulting in them moving within the body
- The organs then experience sudden deceleration when they impact the structures of the body such as the ribcage
- This rapid transfer of energy and rapid deceleration can then cause the internal structures of the body to shear such as the great vessels in the chest

Transfer of energy

Falls from height onto feet

- Faller impacts the ground with their feet
- Impacts on the Calcanei
- The shock wave is sent up through the body
- Potential injuries to the knees where the energy is transferred across the joint space
- Potential injuries to the acetabulum as the thinnest part of the pelvis as energy is transferred up
- Crush injuries possible within the spine especially at thoraco-lumbar and cervico-thoracic junctions
- Potential for high cervical spine injuries
- Basal skull fractures possible

Transfer of energy

237

Blast injuries

Blast injuries occur where there is a rapid decompression or expansion of gas, that is an explosion. There are three moments within a blast injury whereby injury may occur.

- The pressure wave from the blast
  - Can physically throw the patient away from the blast
  - Damage to gas-filled organs, that is the bowel and lungs
  - Gasses will expand in the hollow organs
  - May result in blast lung
- Flying debris
  - Unpredictable injuries
- Patient being thrown against other objects
  - Unpredictable trauma pattern and the patient may be some distance from their starting position

References and Further Reading

Banks, D.E. (2015). *Combat Anaesthesia: The First 24 Hours*. Houston: Borden Institute.

Greaves, I. and Porter, K. (2007). *Oxford Handbook of Pre-Hospital Care*. Oxford: Oxford University Press.

Gregory, P. and Ward, A. (2010). *Sanders' Paramedic Textbook*. Edinburgh: Mosby Elsevier.

Nutbeam, T. and Boylan, M. (2013). *ABC of Prehospital Emergency Medicine*. Chichester: Wiley.

Ridpath, I. (2012). *A Dictionary of Astronomy*. 2nd Revised Edition. Oxford: Oxford University Press.

Royal College of Surgeons of Edinburgh (2019). *Generic Core Material: Prehospital Emergency Care Course*. Edinburgh: Royal College of Surgeons of Edinburgh.

Physiology of trauma

There are a number of physiological considerations in trauma beyond the visible injury. The body's ability to compensate varies due to a number of factors including age and pre-morbid state.

Lethal triad

The lethal triad is a term used to describe factors that increase the risk of mortality following trauma. Each element can worsen others.

- Hypothermia
  - Reduces ability to clot effectively
  - Affects normal metabolism resulting in worsened acidosis
- Acidosis
  - Reduces ability to clot effectively
  - Altered metabolism and oxygen-carrying
- Coagulopathy
  - Increased blood loss
  - Increased mortality

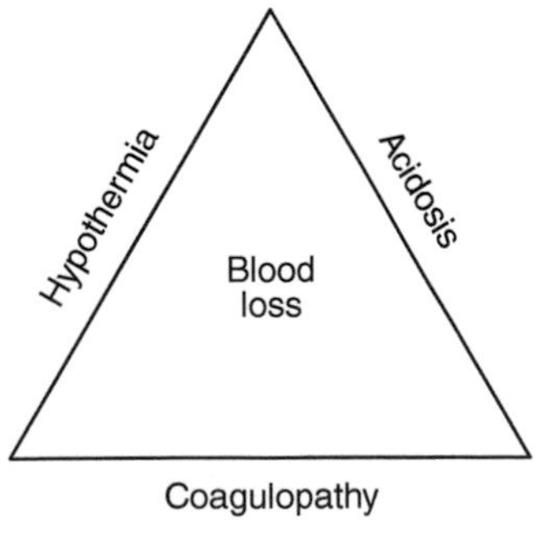

Figure 13.1   Lethal triad.

This demonstrates the pertinence of ensuring the trauma patient is kept warm, oxygenated and haemorrhage addressed as a priority.

Crush syndrome

- Arises following prolonged impingement of vascular supply
- May be as a result of industrial trauma or secondary to simple trauma such as a 'long lie'
- May also occur following compartment syndrome
- Muscle and tissue distal to the impinged vascular supply becomes ischaemic
- Ischemia results in cell death and cell break down (lysis)
- Lysis releases intracellular potassium into circulation
  - Intracellular potassium is a much higher concentration than systemic
- As well as potassium other systemically toxic chemicals are released in the tissue breakdown (rhabdomyolysis)
- Due to vascular impingement, the hyperkalaemia is isolated to the affected area
- If the area is perfused rapidly without intervention may result in a systemic hyperkalaemia
- Hyperkalaemia can cause cardiac arrest
- Specific management for crush injuries should be as per your local policies

239

The body's response to trauma

There are three main drivers for the body's response to trauma, pain, blood loss and inflammation.
Pain

- Relays message to brain of injury
- Tachycardia
- Stimulates the release of adrenaline and cortisol
- Central nervous system innervation

Blood loss

- Reduced venous return to the right heart (reduced preload)
- Detected by baroreceptors
- Tachycardia
- Vasoconstriction
- Fluid retention in the kidneys
- Vasoconstriction
- Stimulates the release of stores

Inflammation

- Immune system response
- Inflammatory mediators released systemically
- Vasodilatation

Altered physiological states

There are occasions whereby the patient may not mount a typical response to trauma and may 'mask' or otherwise alter the symptoms of the bodies normal mechanisms. The word mask is in quotation marks as the signs may be visible but may require further investigation or consideration.

Medication

- Beta-blockers
  - Patient's may not be able to mount a tachycardia response
  - May not fall within typical triage tools
  - Reduced ability to respond to hypotension
- Anti-hypertensives
  - Reduce the body's ability to respond to hypotension
  - May present with more profound hypotension from relatively low mechanism trauma
  - Hypotension in trauma increases mortality

Fitness

- Patients at peak fitness especially athletes will have an altered baseline
- Athletes may have very low resting heart rates and strong cardiac contractility
- As a result, a 'normal' heart rate may be the same as a profound tachycardia
- A 'normal' heart rate in an athlete should be considered a sign of trauma

Elderly

- Reduced physiological ability to respond to trauma
- Altered baseline physiology
- May be taking medications that otherwise affect their ability to respond to trauma
- Low mechanisms may result in major trauma injuries

Children

- Signs may be mistaken for 'normal' physiology
- May be non-verbal
- Practitioner inexperience

Quick Questions

1. What makes up the triad of death for trauma?
2. How do you calculate kinetic energy?
3. Why is this important?

References and Further Reading

Association of Ambulance Chief Executives (2019). *JRCALC Clinical Guidelines*. Bridgewater: Class Professional Publishing.

Banks, D.E. (2015). *Combat Anaesthesia: The First 24 Hours*. Houston: Borden Institute.

Gonzalez, D. (2005). Crush syndrome. *Critical Care Medicine* **33** (supp. 1): 34–41.

Greaves, I. and Porter, K. (2007). *Oxford Handbook of Pre-Hospital Care*. Oxford: Oxford University Press.

Gregory, P. and Ward, A. (2010). *Sanders' Paramedic Textbook*. Edinburgh: Mosby Elsevier.

Nickson, C. (2019). Crush syndrome. LITFL. https://litfl.com/crush-syndrome/ (accessed 24 August 2020).

Norris, T.L. (2018). *Porth's Pathophysiology: Concepts of Altered Health States*, 10e. Philidelphia: Wolters Kluwer.

Nutbeam, T. and Boylan, M. (2013). *ABC of Prehospital Emergency Medicine*. Chichester: Wiley.

Royal College of Surgeons of Edinburgh (2019). *Generic Core Material: Prehospital Emergency Care Course*. Edinburgh: Royal College of Surgeons of Edinburgh.

Penetrating and blunt force trauma

This section will look in a little more detail at some of the forms of a trauma you may encounter.

Penetrating

- May be low velocity
  - Knives and blades etc
- May be high velocity
  - Rifles and firearms
- Injury may be directly associated with the penetrated area
  - Direct wounds to organs or cavities especially with bladed articles
- Affected areas may be indirectly affected
  - Cavitation injury from high-velocity firearms
- Consider entry and exit
  - Gives an idea of the potential path of the injury and underlying structures
  - Be aware of the absence of exit wounds
- Path of injury may not be clear
  - The stab wound to the abdomen may have been upwards and with sufficient length, blade may have entered the thoracic cavity
- May be secondary to the initial insult
  - The patient may have been thrown against a sharp implement or fallen onto a sharp point causing both blunt and penetrating injuries
- Imbedded articles should not be removed pre-hospitally
  - May be occluding blood loss and removal may initiate uncontrollable haemorrhage
- Penetrating injuries to the back may cause lung or chest injuries
  - Just because it is the back does not negate the fact it may be thoracic

Blunt

- May be direct
  - Body impacting with an object
- May be indirect
  - Deceleration injuries
- May involve more than one system or organ
- Organs susceptible to injury from ligaments normally responsible for their anatomical support for example
  - Ligamentum arteriosis (aorta)
  - Falciform ligament (liver)
- Rib fractures may be simple or flail
  - Flail segments whereby the rib is broken in more than on location
- May cause penetrating injury
  - Blunt force trauma to the chest may cause rib fractures that result in cardiac injury although this is rare

Blood loss

- Notoriously difficult to estimate
- May be internal and external
- May have been soaked into surrounding areas or clothing
- Preference should be for blood or blood products following substantial blood loss

241

- Physiology may not present until late after the blood loss
- Typical shock models do not always apply in acute trauma

Critical care

- Penetrating injury may result in cardiac tamponade
- Patients may present awake and talking and then become unresponsive and present with cardiac arrest
- Critical care teams and appropriate receiving units may be able to provide thoracotomy to relieve cardiac tamponade
- Critical care teams may be able to provide thoracotomies where typical needle thoracocentesis is insufficient in relieving tension pneumothorax
- Critical care teams typically carry blood or blood products and are well drilled in the provision of pre-hospital blood
- Blunt force trauma may be complex and require intervention from the critical care team
- Polytrauma may benefit from early intervention and stabilisation to facilitate admission direct to major trauma centre
- Critical care teams will carry an array of analgesic options that may be more suitable for the altered physiology seen with trauma

References and Further Reading

Banks, D.E. (2015). *Combat Anaesthesia: The First 24 Hours*. Houston: Borden Institute.

Bose, P., Regan, F., and Paterson-Brown, S. (2006). Improving the accuracy of estimated blood loss at obstetric haemorrhage using clinical reconstructions. *International Journal of Obstetrics and Gynecology* **113** (8): 919–924.

Greaves, I. and Porter, K. (2007). *Oxford Handbook of Pre-Hospital Care*. Oxford: Oxford University Press.

Gregory, P. and Ward, A. (2010). *Sanders' Paramedic Textbook*. Edinburgh: Mosby Elsevier.

Nutbeam, T. and Boylan, M. (2013). *ABC of Prehospital Emergency Medicine*. Chichester: Wiley.

Royal College of Surgeons of Edinburgh (2019). *Generic Core Material: Prehospital Emergency Care Course*. Edinburgh: Royal College of Surgeons of Edinburgh.

Spinal trauma

This section will look at the decision tools regarding spinal immobilisation.

Head injuries

- Aim to reduce secondary brain injury
- Early intervention from an anaesthetic capable pre-hospital critical care team
- Discussed in 'Paramedic Anatomy and Physiology – 2'
- Injuries may be subtle

Spinal injuries

- Transection of the spinal cord will result in loss of nervous innervation below that point
- Loss of nervous innervation will result in vasodilatation
- Hypotension may be a result of vasodilatation or haemorrhage
- If hypotensive with suspected spinal injury search for signs of haemorrhage
- Loss of normal feedback mechanisms
- Secondary injury can be prevented by suitable immobilisation mechanisms
- The shift towards self extrication where possible (refer to local policy)

- C-Spine assessment may be done through the NEXUS rules or the Canadian C-Spine rules. These are adapted and incorporated into the JRCALC guidance and local guidelines. Refer to local policy.

Canadian C-spine rules

Any high-risk factor that mandates imaging?

- Age > 65 years
- Paraesthesia in extremities
- Dangerous Mechanism
  - Fall > 3 foot
  - Axial loading, that is diving onto the head
  - High-speed motor accident > 100 km/hr
  - Rollover RTC
  - Ejection from the vehicle following RTC
  - Motorised recreational vehicles
  - Bicycle collisions

> If the answer to any is **YES** the patient requires imaging of their C-Spine.

If no high-risk factor identified: Any low-risk factor that allows safe assessment of a range of movement?

- Simple rear-end collision
  - Not pushed into oncoming traffic
  - Not hit by a large goods vehicle or bus
  - Not a roll-over
  - Not hit by a high-speed vehicle
- The sitting position in ED
- Ambulatory at any time
- Delayed onset of neck pain
  - That is, not immediate onset neck pain
- Absence of midline c-spine tenderness

> If the answer is **NO** the patient requires imaging of their C-Spine.

If the mechanism falls within the low-risk group and does not have any high-risk factors assess a range of movement.

Range of movement

- Actively able to rotate their neck through 45°

If the patient is able to complete this then there is no indication for C-Spine imaging

> If the patient **IS NOT** able to rotate their neck they require imaging of their C-Spine.

NEXUS C-spine rules

- No posterior midline C-Spine tenderness
- No evidence of intoxication
- The normal level of alertness
- No focal neurological deficit
- No painful distracting injuries

> If these criteria are met, there is no indication for C-Spine imaging.

References and Further Reading

Bersten, A.D. and Handy, J.M. (2018). *Oh's Intensive Care Manual*. Edinburgh: Elsevier.

Greaves, I. and Porter, K. (2007). *Oxford Handbook of Pre-Hospital Care*. Oxford: Oxford University Press.

Nickson, C. (2019). Cerebral perfusion pressure in TBI. LITFL. https://litfl.com/cerebral-perfusion-pressure-in-tbi/ (accessed 21 July 2020).

Nickson, C. (2019). Traumatic Brain Injury (TBI) overview. LITFL. https://litfl.com/traumatic-brain-injury-tbi-overview/ (accessed 21 July 2020).

Nutbeam, T. and Boylan, M. (2013). *ABC of Prehospital Emergency Medicine*. Chichester: Wiley.

Pinto, V.L., Tadi, P., and Adeyinka, A. (2020). Increased intracranial pressure. StatPearls. https://www.ncbi.nlm.nih.gov/books/NBK482119/ (accessed 21 July 2020).

Royal College of Surgeons of Edinburgh (2019). *Generic Core Material: Prehospital Emergency Care Course*. Edinburgh: Royal College of Surgeons of Edinburgh.

Saragiotto B.T., Maher C.G., Lin C.C. *et al.* (2018) Canadian C-spine rule and the National Emergency X-Radiography Utilization Study (NEXUS) for detecting clinically important cervical spine injury following blunt trauma. *Cochrane Database of Systematic Reviews*. 1–11. https://www.cochranelibrary.com/cdsr/doi/10.1002/14651858.CD012989/full (accessed 24 August 2020).

Steill, I.G. et al. (2001). The Canadian C-spine rule for radiography in alert and stable trauma patients. *JAMA* **286** (15): 1841–1848.

Steill, I.G., Wells, G.A., Vandemheen, V.A. et al. (2009). Implementation of the Canadian C-spine rule: a prospective 12 centre cluster randomised trial. *British Medical Journal* **339**: 1841–1848.

Tortora, G.J. and Derrickson, B.H. (2017). *Tortora's Principles of Anatomy and Physiology*, 15e. Chichester: Wiley.

Vaillancourt, C., Steil, I.G., Beaudoin, T. et al. (2009). The out-of-hospital validation of the Canadian C-spine rule by paramedics. *Annals of Emergency Medicine* **54** (5): 663–671.

Fractures and burns

This section will look at conditions affecting the long bones as well as a little more information on the management of serious burns injury.

Types of fracture

There are a number of ways to describe fractures; the first is whether the fracture (break) is open or closed.

Open

- The broken bone has caused a rupture in the skin layer
- The bone may have retracted back below the skin layer before the arrival of EMS
- Can be confused with a fracture with overlying laceration not caused by the bone and where the bone has not come into contact with open-air
- Blood loss may be internal or external
- High risk of infection to the bone
  - Refer to local policy for treatment with antibiotics

Closed

- Bone has not been exposed to open air
- Fracture is contained within the tissues
- Blood loss may be internal

Threatened

- Bone is pressing against the skin
- Risk of the bone piercing the skin layer
- May be whiteish in appearance where there is the restricted blood supply

When discussing bone fractures consideration should be given to the type of deformity that is seen. Namely, whether the bone structures have been displaced.

Displaced

- Bone has been misshapen from normal anatomical alignment
- Greater chance of increased blood loss

Non-displaced

- Bones remain in normal anatomical alignment despite injury
- Lesser chance of significant blood loss

Once the fracture has been described as either open or closed and displaced or non-displaced there is classification of fractures. Although these will require imaging thus should give you an idea of the types you may encounter, as not all will be grossly deformed.

Transverse

- Bisects the bone at 90° (across the bone)

Linear

- Fractured along the length of the bone

Oblique

- Bisects the bone at an angle

Spiral

- Bone has been twisted around a breakpoint resulting in a spiral-shaped break

Greenstick

- Incomplete fracture from bending
- Most commonly seen in children

Comminuted

- Bone is 'shattered' into multiple pieces

These are just some of the main types of fractures although there are many more descriptors used within the hospital.

Le Fort fractures

Le Fort fractures describe transverse fractures of the face and skull. They are separated into Le Fort I, Le Fort II and Le Fort III fractures. These typically occur from high-speed facila impacts into blunt objects.

Le Fort I

- Separation of the hard palate from the upper maxilla
- The fracture occurs just above the floor of the nose

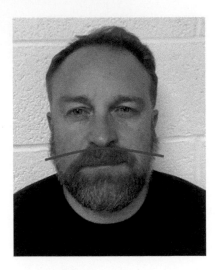

Figure 13.2   Le Fort 1.

Le Fort II

- Fractures transverse the nasal bones
- The fracture extends through anterior-medial orbit and orbital floor

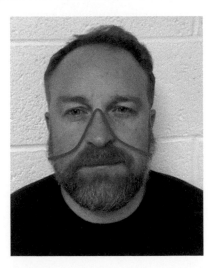

Figure 13.3   Le Fort 2.

Le Fort III

- Separation of the maxilla from the skull base
- Extends through both orbits
- Highest level of Le Fort Fracture

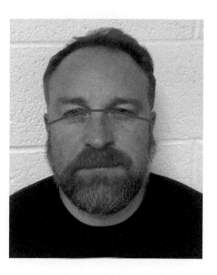

Figure 13.4   Le Fort 3.

Management of burns

In 'Practical Skills for Paramedics – 1', we covered the assessment of burn size and some of the basics of managing burns injuries, this section will look at the resuscitation of burns injuries.

Assess the airway for high-risk signs

- Burns to the face and/or mouth
- Soot in or around the mouth
- Burnt nasal hairs
- Burnt facial hairs
- Stridor and/or hoarse voice
- Cough
- Beware of the patients asleep in a burning house who may have breathed in hot gasses or smoke for a prolonged period of time

Fluid resuscitation may be required if the patient has extensive burns (>20% in adults or >10% in children and the elderly – although refer to local policy for local variation).

- Assess burn surface area
- Erythema excluded
- Fluid resuscitation (Modified Parkland Formula)

Modified Parkland Formula

$4 \times$ (% of Total Body Surface Area Burnt $\times$ Patient's weight in Kg) = Total 24-hour fluid in mL

50% given over the initial eight hours

50% given over the remaining 16 hours

References and Further Reading

Banks, D.E. (2015). *Combat Anaesthesia: The First 24 Hours*. Houston: Borden Institute.

Bersten, A.D. and Handy, J.M. (2018). *Oh's Intensive Care Manual*. Edinburgh: Elsevier.

Bowden, G., McNally, M.A., Thomas, S.R.Y.W. et al. (2010). *Oxford Handbook of Orthopaedics and Trauma*. Oxford: Oxford University Press.

Funk, G. (2017). Facial fracture management handbook. University of Iowa. https://medicine.uiowa.edu/iowaprotocols/content/facial-fracture-management-handbook (accessed 24 August 2020).

Greaves, I. and Porter, K. (2007). *Oxford Handbook of Pre-Hospital Care*. Oxford: Oxford University Press.

Gregory, P. and Ward, A. (2010). *Sanders' Paramedic Textbook*. Edinburgh: Mosby Elsevier.

Mehta, M. and Tudor, G.J. (2020). Parkland formula. StatPearls. https://www.ncbi.nlm.nih.gov/books/NBK537190/ (accessed 25 August 2020).

Nutbeam, T. and Boylan, M. (2013). *ABC of Prehospital Emergency Medicine*. Chichester: Wiley.

Royal College of Surgeons of Edinburgh (2019). *Generic Core Material: Prehospital Emergency Care Course*. Edinburgh: Royal College of Surgeons of Edinburgh.

Thom, D. (2017). Appraising current methods for preclinical calculation of burn size - a pre-hospital perspective. *Burns* **43** (1): 127–136.

Traumatic cardiac arrest

Although thankfully in UK civilian practice traumatic cardiac arrest is a rare event first responders may still encounter. Traumatic cardiac arrest has a poor survival and even if ROSC is achieved has poor outcomes. Early maximal treatment is currently recommended and early assistance from pre-hospital critical care teams.

HOTT principles

The management of traumatic cardiac arrest currently involves aggressive and early correction of the reversible causes for traumatic cardiac arrest. These are referred to as the HOTT principles

H – Hypovolaemia
O – Oxygen (Hypoxia)
T – Tension pneumothorax
T – Tamponade

Hypovolaemia

- Apply tourniquets if required
- Draw limbs to length and normal anatomical alignment
  - Reduces space in which to bleed
  - Splint as able
- Apply pelvic binder
- IV/IO access
- Blood transfusion
- Fluids as per local policy, preference is for blood or blood products

Oxygen

- Airway management
  - Simple methods
  - Simple adjuncts acceptable
  - A role for iGel as quick and simple and the BVM can then be handed to a non-skilled bystander/police officer/firefighter to perform ventilation

- Maximise oxygenation
- High flow oxygen

Tension pneumothorax

- Decompression
  - Needle thoracocentesis
  - Finger thoracostomies if trained and governed to do so

Tamponade

- Critical care teams can consider a resuscitative thoracotomy if indicated

Drugs

There is little evidence to support the role of adrenaline in traumatic cardiac arrest

249

CPR

CPR in traumatic cardiac arrest may be contentious but guidelines allow for the delayed initiation of CPR in order to facilitate rapid correction of reversible causes (HOTT).

Patients may gain ROSC from implementing the HOTT principles and receiving a bolus of blood/fluid prior to CPR being started.

Refer to local policy.

Quick Questions

1. What are the key principles of HOTT?
2. Describe a comminuted fracture
3. What makes up the NEXUS C-Spine rules?

References and Further Reading

Banks, D.E. (2015). *Combat Anaesthesia: The First 24 Hours*. Houston: Borden Institute.

Greaves, I. and Porter, K. (2007). *Oxford Handbook of Pre-Hospital Care*. Oxford: Oxford University Press.

Lockey, D.J., Lyon, R.M., and Davies, G.E. (2012). Development of a simple algorithm to guide the effective management of traumatic cardiac arrest. *Resuscitation* **84**: 738–742.

Nutbeam, T. and Boylan, M. (2013). *ABC of Prehospital Emergency Medicine*. Chichester: Wiley.

Royal College of Surgeons of Edinburgh (2018). Consensus statement: management of traumatic cardiac arrest. RCSEd. https://fphc.rcsed.ac.uk/media/2577/tca-submission-oct-2018.pdf (accessed 24 August 2020).

Royal College of Surgeons of Edinburgh (2019). *Generic Core Material: Prehospital Emergency Care Course*. Edinburgh: Royal College of Surgeons of Edinburgh.

Smith, J.E., Rickard, A., and Wise, D. (2015). Traumatic cardiac arrest. *Journal of the Royal Society of Medicine* **108** (1): 11–16.

The Royal College of Emergency Medicine (2019). Traumatic cardiac arrest in adults: best practice guideline. RCEM. https://www.rcem.ac.uk/docs/RCEM%20Guidance/RCEM_Traumatic%20cardiac%20arrest_Sept%202019%20FINAL.pdf (accessed 24 August 2020).

14

Pharmacology – 3

Contents

This section will look to build on the topics already covered and apply them to altered health states you may encounter. This will cover the basics of pharmacology for patients with liver dysfunction and kidney dysfunction as well as the elderly.

Further pharmacokinetics

Further to what has already been covered, there are a few extra points to consider
Bioavailability

- Amount of drug that is available to the systemic circulation
- Not related to the efficacy of the medication
- IV medication has 100% bioavailability

Plasma binding

- Drugs are typically inactive when protein-bound within the plasma
  - Free molecules (unbound) can exert their therapeutic effect
- Protein binding is dependant not only on the drug but the physiological state of the body
- Factors affecting binding will affect the drug's efficacy
  - Can increase or decrease drug efficacy
  - May result in toxic plasma concentrations
- Drugs can compete for the same plasma protein binding sites
  - The competition will create a more free molecule of one drug to exert its effect

The Paramedic Revision Guide, First Edition. David W. Thom.
© 2021 John Wiley & Sons Ltd. Published 2021 by John Wiley & Sons Ltd.

Ionisation

- Lipophilic cell membrane allows passage of ionised (free molecule) drug
- pKa is achieved when 50% of the drug is ionised
- Affected by the systemic environment
- Local or systemic Acidosis may increase or decrease the efficacy of the drug
  - Inflammation at a wound site may decrease the efficacy of Lidocaine

Cytochrome P450 (CYP450)

- Group of Liver enzymes
- Involved in the metabolism of drugs
- Some drugs share the same subgroup and therefore will interact
  - Increased or decreased metabolism of one or other drug if given concurrently
- Activating additional subgroups may assist in the metabolism of other drugs
  - Caffeine as an example
  - Some 'anti-dotes' may work by acting upon the CYP450 pathways

251

Renal failure

Renal failure can affect pharmacology in a number of ways; here are some considerations when treating a patient with renal failure or dysfunction.

- Consider what medications the patient is already taking
- Renal excretion reduces with age
  - Drugs administered will stay within the body for a longer time
- Renal failure is a spectrum
  - Patients may have a chronic low-level impairment or be on long term dialysis and everything in between
- Renal failure can be acute
  - May be a new issue arising from the presenting condition such as rhabdomyolysis or hypotension especially in susceptible patients
- Consider the indication for medications
- Consider any cautions on the administration that may surround the medication
- Renal failure may be concurrent with other system dysfunction such as cardiac failure
- Avoid sedative drugs or drugs that are largely renal excreted where possible
- Patient's may be on a fluid restriction
  - Consider the volume in which medicines are being administered and clearly document
- Patient's may be on a sodium restriction
- Dose reduction may be required
- Always best to start with a low dose and increase the dose intervals
- If in doubt seek senior advice

Liver failure

As with renal failure, there are a number of ways that liver failure or dysfunction may affect the drugs you administer.

- Drugs may be less well absorbed if they require bile salts for absorption
  - Lipid soluble drugs

- Liver failure may create new fluid compartments
  - Ascites
  - Oedema
  - Water-soluble drugs may be distributed into these spaces
- Chronic liver failure may result in reduced plasma protein levels
  - Reduced protein binding sites
  - Increased free molecules
  - Potential for increased efficacy of medications beyond expected
- Reduced or delays metabolism of medications
  - Medications may remain active within the body for longer than expected
  - Pro-drugs may take longer to be metabolised or not be converted at all
- Patients may require a dose reduction
- Always best to start with a low dose and increase the dose intervals
- If in doubt seek senior advice

Elderly

There are some specific considerations for medications in the elderly as well as some overlapping themes.

- The acute presentation may be as a result of current medications
- Actions of common drugs may be unpredictable in the elderly
- Reduced number of and efficacy of drug receptors
- Increased affinity for opiates and benzodiazepines
- Lower physiological reserve to cope with the effects of medications
  - Expected or adverse
- Drugs will have a narrower therapeutic window
- Uncertain absorption of oral medications
- Delayed gastric emptying may delay the onset of oral medication
- Variable 1st pass metabolism
- The decrease in plasma protein therefore reduced protein binding of medications
- Changes in distribution due to body fat and muscle variations
- Reduced hepatic (liver) metabolism
- Decreased renal excretion therefore drugs may stay within the body for longer
- Smaller volumes of fluid may be required to cause fluid overload states
- Consider the necessity for medication before administering
- Dose reduction may be required
- Always best to start with a low dose and increase the dose intervals
- If in doubt seek senior advice

Children

- Varied gastric absorption and emptying dependant on age
- IM Medications have variable and unpredictable absorption
  - Reduced muscle mass
- May have underlying health conditions
- Varying distribution of medications
- Immature hepatic metabolism in younger children
  - Older children may have greater hepatic function than adults
  - Variable

- The increased half-life of medications
- Increased plasma concentration of medication
- Variable excretion of medication
- Most medications are off-label for use in children

Questions

1. True or false
   a. Drugs are typically inert when they are plasma bound
   b. A pro-drug enters the body in a from that can immediately take effect
   c. Liver failure creates new fluid compartments.
2. How might liver failure alter the person's response to a medication?
3. Why might a dose reduction be required in the elderly?

References and Further Reading

Nutall, D. and Rutt-Howard, J. (2019). *The Textbook of Non-Medical Prescribing*, 3e. Chichester: Wiley Blackwell.

Ritter, J.M., Fower, R., Henderson, G. et al. (2019). *Rang and Dale's Pharmacology*, 9e. Edinburgh: Elsevier.

Royal Pharmaceutical Society (2020). *BNF: 80*. London: BMJ Group, RCPCH Publications Ltd and the Royal Pharmaceutical Society of Great Britain.

Tortora, G.J. and Derrickson, B.H. (2017). *Tortora's Principles of Anatomy and Physiology*, 15e. Chichester: Wiley.

Waugh, A. and Grant, A. (2018). *Ross and Wilson Anatomy and Physiology*. Edinburgh: Elsevier.

Whalen, K. (2018). *Pharmacology*, 7e. Philidelphia: Wolters Kluwer.

15

Research and evidence-based practice – 3

Contents

This section will look to build further on the previous chapters and gain further insight into how to interpret research in practice.

Additional research terms

Table 15.1   Research terms.

Research term	Explanation	Example
Publication bias	Positive results are more likely to be published than negative	Studies that are intended to show a benefit in treatment such as one drug over another may find that there is no benefit or in fact the study drug is worse than current options. In these cases, researchers are less likely to publish the findings resulting in only positive studies being published, which may result in a skewed data set when compared to larger non-published databases.
Journal bias	A reader pre-judges the credibility of a paper by the journal it is published in	A reader may be lulled into a false sense of security if an article is published in a prestigious or high impact journal and/or may dismiss research that has been published in lower impact journals.

The Paramedic Revision Guide, First Edition. David W. Thom.
© 2021 John Wiley & Sons Ltd. Published 2021 by John Wiley & Sons Ltd.

Table 15.1 (Continued)

Research term	Explanation	Example
Odds ratio (OR)	Association between an event and an outcome	Thus, looks to see the relative odds of a particular outcome given a particular event or treatment compared to both the outcome not occurring at all and also the outcome occurring without the event in the first place. To simplify this further lets take the example of if the outcome is sickness, and the event is the administration of morphine. We will use a random set of numbers that do not apply to any research but demonstrate the point.

<table>
<tr><td></td><td>**Sickness**</td><td>**No sickness**</td></tr>
<tr><td>Morphine</td><td>10 (a)</td><td>4 (b)</td></tr>
<tr><td>No morphine</td><td>5 (c)</td><td>3 (d)</td></tr>
</table>

The odds ratio is then calculated as:

$$ad/bc$$

In this instance, the odds ratio would be 1.5

An odds ratio (OR) of greater than 1 indicates an increased occurrence of the outcome following treatment. If the OR is less than 1, there is a decreased occurrence or the treatment may be protective.

However, it does not mean that the outcome is 1.5 times more likely to occur it simply provides a ratio.

The OR does not replace the confidence interval or the P value, and these will give you an idea of the statistical significance of the results.

Research term	Explanation	Example
Fragility index (FI)	The amount of patients in a study that would have needed to got a different result in order to not achieve a statistically significant result.	If a study achieved a positive result and got a P value of <0.05 this would be considered statistically significant. However, if the study only required 1 patient to have not had a positive result for the P value to go above 0.05 (and therefore not statistically significant) the fragility index would be 1. The lower the Fragility index the less patients that would need to have had a different result to affect the results.
Intention to treat analysis (ITT)	All patients that get randomised are included for analysis despite any deviations in protocol	Occasionally in studies once a patient has been randomised into a group they may receive a treatment that is not included in the study protocol. By normal analysis, these patients are excluded along with any patient's that may be a lot to follow-up or withdrew, etc The benefit of this is meant to replicate the real-world scenarios faced by clinicians every day and not just within rigid protocols and should reduce type 1 error and bias from incomplete data sets. However, there is an increased risk of type 2 error and protocol violations may reduce the validity of the results. Results from an ITT may appear different to standard analysis.

255

Performing a search

During your training and career, it will be necessary to search for research papers or perform a search on a specific topic. This section will cover a few of the basics to help you get the best results.

Most institutions will have access to designated search engines for performing a search. A standard online search engine will not have the specificity to pull papers from journals. A typical example of this is the 'MEDLINE' database. Other search engines such as 'PubMed', 'CINAHL' and 'Google Scholar'.

There are a few ways to help narrow your search so that you can get the best out of the search engines.

Boolean Operators, Truncation and wildcard searching:

These are used to help add additional information to the search or actively exclude, they are 'AND', 'OR' and 'NOT'. They are fairly self-explanatory but to give an example of how they are used.

Often you will want to limit the search to papers relating to Paramedic so that you are not overloaded with unrelated papers. For example, if you wanted to look at the use of analgesia by paramedics you might search: Analgesia AND Paramedic. This would provide you with papers that mention both analgesia and Paramedics.

However, some papers may be more general and look at analgesia across all clinicians in the pre-hospital setting, therefore you would want to include the term pre-hospital as well. This would be achieved by Analgesia AND (Paramedic OR Pre-Hospital). When using multiple search terms these are described in parenthesis.

Some papers may use different acceptable spellings for the terms, this is especially important for hyphenation as well as Anglo American spelling differences. In these cases, it may be useful to use a wildcard search. In this case, the hyphen is replaced with a question mark (?) which means the search will reveal both 'Pre-Hospital and Prehospital'. This is achieved by Analgesia AND (Paramedic OR Pre?hospital).

In some instances, you may want to use the start of a word as the root of your search but allow variation. For example, in some papers, you may see Paramedic practice referred to as Paramedicine. In which case, if you wanted to search for Paramedic, Paramedics and Paramedicine the easiest way to do this is by using a truncation search by using an asterisk (*) at the end of the root you want to search. In this instance, it would be would be: Analgesia AND (Paramedic* OR pre?hospital).

Finally, if you had a particular interest in a specific area of prehospital analgesia, such as medical conditions causing pain, you may wish to actively exclude a portion of papers. Typically, analgesia would focus on trauma so if you wanted to exclude these at the search you could utilise the NOT function. For example, in this case, it would be: Analgesia AND (Paramedic* OR pre?hospital) NOT trauma.

Prior to performing your search you should determine, using the PICO format covered previously, the search terms you wish to use. In order to gain the maximum amount of papers from the databases, you can generate alternative search terms using synonyms.

For example, if you wanted to see if using a set protocol to provide a rapid sequence induction reduces the risk you might structure your PICO like this:

Table 15.2 Example PICO question.

P – Population	Adult patients requiring emergency rapid sequence induction (RSI)
I – Intervention	Use of a protocol
C – Comparison	Standard practice (operator choice)
O – Outcome	Reduction in adverse incidents

From this, you can structure your synonyms and decide on your Boolean operators. For example:

Table 15.3 Example synonym table and Boolean search strategy.

PICO descriptor	Chosen term		Synonyms
Population (1)	1a) Rapid sequence induction	**OR**	1b) Rapid sequence intubation 1c) Emergency an?esthe* 1d) RSI
AND			
Intervention (2)	2a) Protocol	**OR**	2b) Standard operating procedure* 2c) SOP 2d) Checklist*
AND			
Comparison (3)	3a) Standard practice	**OR**	3b) Operator choice 3c) Personal preference 3d) Current practice
AND			
Outcome (4)	4a) Adverse incidents	**OR**	4b) Adverse events 4c) Complication 4d) Mortality

The PICO term and the synonyms can be searched concurrently using the OR operator prior to the AND. For example, this would be: (rapid sequence induction OR rapid sequence intubation OR emergency an?ethe* OR rsi) AND (protocol OR standard operating procedure* OR sop OR checklist*) AND (standard practice OR operator choice OR personal preference OR current practice) AND (adverse incidents OR adverse events OR complication OR mortality).

Although this search seems lengthy and wordy by doing it in this manner, it collates all the papers into a single list and means you don't have to do multiple searches and risk multiple duplicate papers.

Applying inclusion and exclusion criteria:

Once you have performed your search you will, usually, still have a large volume of papers returned. This is where the inclusion and exclusion criteria are useful to help narrow the search to the most relevant papers. Often this will include limiting the age of the papers to the last 5–10 years to make sure you are reading the most up-to-date research. However, some research is deemed 'Seminal' whereby the age is irrelevant as it is the main paper on this field.

Other factors that might be used to exclude papers are being published in a journal or magazine that is not peer-reviewed as the peer review process is designed to ensure a degree of credibility. Papers not available in native languages are usually excluded at the undergraduate level due to online translation services being unreliable and professional translation expensive. If, however, you are fluent in another language it may be acceptable to use papers in that language depending on your institution. However, if using a foreign paper, you should assess its relevance to the setting you wish to apply as infrastructure, epidemiology and clinical variation may affect the interpretation and application of results. Availability of papers may result in exclusion as if you are unable to access the full article you should not interpret the results from the abstract, as they may not give the full picture.

Quick Questions

1. What is publication bias?
2. How do you search with truncation?

References and Further Reading

Bland, J.M. and Altman, D.G. (2000). The odds ratio. *BMJ* **320**: 1468.

DeVito, N.J. and Goldacre, B. (2019). Catalogue of bias: publication bias. *BMJ Evidence-Based Medicine* **24**: 53–54.

Fergusson, D., Aaron, S.D., Guyatt, G. et al. (2002). Post-randomisation exclusions: the intention to treat principle and excluding patients from analysis. *BMJ* **325**: 652–654.

Mathieu, S. (2017). Fragility index. TBL. www.thebottomline.org.uk/blog/ebm/fragility-index/ (accessed 04 September 2020).

Polit, D.F. and Beck, C.T. (2013). *Essentials of Nursing Research: Appraising Evidence for Nursing Practice*, 8e. Philadelphia: Lippincott Williams and Wilkins.

Answers

Page 4

1. Check these yourself against the previous pages
2. **a.** Lateral
   b. Inferior
   c. Anterior
   d. Cephalic
   e. Distal
3. Supine
4. Midsagittal
5. Flexion
6. Right inguinal or right iliac depending on the preference of term
7. Hypotension (we will cover this later)
8. Neck of femur fracture

Page 7

1. False, the smooth endoplasmic reticulum synthesis lipids
2. True
3. False, the movement of water is known as osmosis
4. False, human cells have a membrane whereas plant cells will have a wall
5. False, the tail is hydrophobic

Page 12

1. **a.** Saltatory
   b. Control centres, effectors
   c. Efferent
2. **a.** False, this is negative feedback – if the body temperature rises the body will try and reduce it by normal mechanisms
   b. False, the nucleus is within the cell body
   c. True
   d. False, although neurotransmitters are reabsorbed the message is only sent one way
3. Oligodendrocytes
4. Warming the patient up

The Paramedic Revision Guide, First Edition. David W. Thom.
© 2021 John Wiley & Sons Ltd. Published 2021 by John Wiley & Sons Ltd.

Page 20

1.   **a.** Outer
     b. Midbrain
     c. Pons Varolii
     d. Medulla Oblongata
     e. Phrenic
     f. Enteric
2.   **a.** False, these are in the Medulla Oblongata
     b. False, the Thalamus is the largest part
     c. True
     d. True
3. Medulla Oblongata
4. Pia mater, Arachnoid mater, Dura mater
5. 80–150 mL

Page 27

1.   **a.** IX, X, and XI
     b. Carina
     c. 1200 mL
     d. Negative
2.   **a.** True
     b. False, the sections are incomplete posteriorly – be careful when reading questions with more than one part. If a question has more than one part that needs to be correct there is a high likelihood that one part will be wrong.
     c. True
3. More oblique angle more likely for objects to fall down
4. Movement of oxygen across the lung membrane

Page 28

1. Nervous control and chemical regulation
2. Hypoxic, anaemic, stagnant, histotoxic
3. Coleslaw is a side dish typically created with shredded cabbage, carrot and mayonnaise
4. Atelectasis
5. Pulmonary ventilation, external respiration, internal respiration

Page 33

1.   **a.** Anti-B
     b. Transportation, protection and regulation
     c. Aorta
2.   **a.** False, slightly alkali
     b. True

    c. False, the pulmonary vein carries oxygenated blood from the lungs to the heart. Be careful with questions that state 'all' or 'none' as there is sometimes an exception. Similarly, with 'always' and 'never' these should make you think twice about any question. Of course, there may be an example with is all just to catch you out

    d. True

3. Artery, Arteriole, Capillary, Venules, Veins
4. During diastole
5. During systole the muscle is contracted and the blood is forcefully ejected into the aorta, when the aortic valve opens it covers the inlet to the coronary circulation to protect the delicate coronary circulation from these pressures. As the muscle relaxes in the diastole, the valve closes and the coronary circulation can fill passively from the blood in the aorta.

Page 38

1. **a.** systole
   b. P wave
2. **a.** True
   b. False, the left ventricle pumps the oxygenated blood to the body
   c. True
3. Between the lungs at approximately the level of T4/5
4. T1-4
5. **a.** Sino-atrial node fires
   b. The impulse spreads across atria
   c. Atrial systole
   d. Atrio-ventricular node holds impulse
   e. The impulse travels down the Bundle of His
   f. The impulse travels into left and right bundle branches
   g. The impulse travels into Purkinje fibres
   h. Ventricular systole
   i. Diastole
6. The point in the cardiac cycle where the ventricles are contracting but all the valves are closed.

Page 47

1. **a.** Acidic
   b. Amino acid
   c. Medulla
   d. Lower
2. **a.** True
   b. False, this is the exocrine portion
   c. False, although it sometimes referred to as two halves
3. Mouth → Oesophagus → Cardiac sphincter → Stomach → Pyloric sphincter → Duodenum → Small intestine → Ascending colon → Transverse colon → Descending colon → Sigmoid colon → Rectum

Page 51

1. **a.** T12 and L3
   b. Ureters
   c. Ureter

2. **a.** False, it is the outer layer
   b. True
3. Adenosine triphosphate
4. **a.** Regulation of blood volume and pressure
   b. Regulation of the concentration of plasma ions
   c. Regulation of blood pH
   d. Conservation of nutrients
5. 6–18

Page 58

1. **a.** Long
   b. 33
   c. Epidermis, dermis and subcutaneous (Hypodermis)
2. **a.** False, these are fixed
   b. True
   c. True
   d. True
3. **a.** Support
   b. Protection
   c. Movement
   d. Mineral homeostasis
   e. Blood cell production
   f. Storage
4. Capacity for fibres to respond to a stimuli
5. Evaporation, conduction, convection
6. Tinning skin, greater sensitivity to sunlight, loss of elasticity

Page 64

1. Scene safety
2. Alert, voice, pain, unresponsive
3. Your personal safety

Page 72

1. Large occiputs and easily kinked trachea mean that the neutral position is the most likely to maintain an open airway
2. 40 mL
3. Tip of the nose to the tragus of the ear
4. Yes – but refer to local policy
5. The 5 P's

Page 74

1. By affecting the conduction in the heart leading to dysrhythmias
2. Early CPR and defibrillation

3. Check for breathing and pulse for up to 10 seconds
4. Check these yourself against the previous pages

Page 81

1. Cover up and check against previous pages
2. Anaphylaxis is a severe and potentially fatal form of a hypersensitivity reaction, which eventually affects all organs usually (but not always) evoked by an antigen.

Page 86

1. Bruising
2. Darker blood continuous flow
3. When direct pressure is not enough to stem the bleeding
4. Avulsion
5. As per the methods mentioned
6. Only affecting the dermis not deeper structures

Page 92

1. The overstretching and/or tearing of a muscle
2. Overlying wound to the fracture causing the bone to be exposed
3. Reduces movement

Page 100

1. Initial injury-causing irreversible damage to the CNS
2. Linear non-displaced fracture of skull bone
3. Can be, but not always, associated with the base of skull fractures

Page 110

1. Absorption, Distribution, Metabolism, Excretion
2. Right drug, the right dose, the right route, and the right time
3. No. A PGD is a legal document that clearly denotes the indications for which a drug can be given by which clinician.
4. Anyone

Page 118

1. a. True
   b. False, it is Immunoglobulin E. Be careful with similar letters in questions
   c. False, it can be associated with other conditions as well. Remember to be cautious if a question has terms like 'always' in it
   d. True

    e. True

    f. False, although glucose is not technically being given to stop the seizure if it is caused by underlying hypoglycaemia then it will correct the metabolic imbalance and may terminate the seizure. Again, and you're probably getting the hang of it now – beware of words like 'never'

2. **a.** Sudden onset and rapid progression of symptoms

    b. Life-threatening airway and/or breathing and/or circulatory problems

    c. Mucosal and/or skin changes

3. **a.** PEFR less than 33% predicted or patient's previous best

    b. Silent chest

    c. Cyanosis

    d. Poor or absent breathing effort

    e. Oxygen saturations less than 92%

    f. Bradycardia

    g. Hypotension

    h. Exhaustion

    i. Coma

4. **a.** Abnormal electrical discharges within the brain

    b. Altered neuron permeability to excitatory ions such as calcium

    c. Relative lack of or ineffective Gamma-Aminobutyric Acid (GABA)

      i. Neuro-regulatory chemical

    d. Hyperpolarisation of the cells resting potential

      i. Increases the resting potential towards the action potential

      ii. Reduced stimulus required to create an action potential

    e. Greatly increased neurological oxygen demand

Page 122

1. Individual high-quality RCT's with narrow confidence intervals

2. Consistent with level 4 evidence **or** extrapolated from level 2 or 3 evidence

3. To describe the weighting of evidence supporting the recommendation

Page 127

1. Consistency and ability to replicate results

2. Population, Intervention, Comparison, Outcome

3. Small scale studies or lab-based assessments

4. Uses numerical data points to inform statistical analysis

Page 133

1. **a.** Patients

    b. Family

    c. Public

    d. Employer

    e. Students

    f. Colleagues

2. Protect the public

3. Above all do no harm

4. Leaving an unresponsive patient at the scene of a major incident to assist other patients with a greater chance of a survivable outcome

Page 140

1. **a.** False, it is negative pressure
   b. False, above 4 L/min tissue damage may occur and it is extremely uncomfortable for the patient
   c. True
   d. True
2. FiO_2, PEEP, Surface area, Diffusion, pH, presence of carbon monoxide or other poisons, hypermetabolic states, perfusion

Page 146

1. **a.** True
   b. True, however, patients may also be profoundly hypotensive and will not have these bounding pulses
   c. False, it will cause an increase. Again, be aware of questions with more than one statement within them that needs to be correct
2. **a.** 1st space – Intra-vascular fluid – The smallest volume of fluid
   b. 2nd space – Intra-cellular fluid – The largest volume of fluid
   c. 3rd space – Interstitial fluid
3. **a.** Increased workload on the ventricles
   b. Increased oxygen demand
   c. Increased effort required to eject blood from the ventricles

Page 149

1. **a.** True
   b. True
   c. False
2. Further cellular damage as a result of the effects of the primary injury
3. **a.** Hypoxia
   i. Hypoventilation as a result of brain injury
   ii. Hypo/hypercapnia
   iii. Hypo/hypertension
   iv. Temperature dysregulation
   v. Glycaemic control anomalies and inability to meet cerebral requirements
   vi. Electrolyte disturbance
   b. Early intervention with airway control, adequate ventilation, calling for the critical care team and normalising physiology as able

Page 152

1. **a.** Hypotension
   b. Hypo/mal-perfusion
   c. Raised intra-abdominal pressures
   d. Acute hypertensive emergencies

2. **a.** ECG changes
   b. Muscle cramps
   c. Arrhythmias including Torsades des Pointes
   d. Heart failure
   e. Further reabsorption of sodium and water
   f. Potassium and hydrogen secreted into the distal tubule
3. **a.** Further reabsorption of sodium and water
   b. Potassium and hydrogen secreted into the distal tubule

Page 161

1. 64.4 mL/min
2. 45 mm (Yellow)
3. **a.** Proximal fracture in the target bone
   b. Previous orthopaedic surgical intervention at or near the target site
      i. Joint replacements are NOT target sites
   c. Previous IO needle insertion in target bone within 48 hours
   d. Infection overlying target site
   e. Inability to locate landmarks for insertion

Page 169

1. **a.** Lips
   b. Teeth
   c. Tongue
   d. Hard palate
   e. Soft palate
   f. Uvula
   g. Posterior wall
   h. Epiglottis
2. Rescue oxygenation for paediatrics in the event of failed airway management, including simple methods, resulting in the inability to oxygenate the patient.
3. **a.** 2nd intercostal space, mid-clavicular line
      OR
   b. 4th/5th intercostal space mid-axillary line

Page 198

1. **a.** False, they are associated with hyperglycaemia
   b. True
   c. True
2. **a.** Muscle rigidity
   b. Confusion
   c. Slow and/or slurred speech
   d. Reduced blood pressure
   e. Arrhythmia

3. **a.** Maintain airway patency
   b. High flow oxygen therapy
   c. Fluid therapy in line with local policy
   d. Immediate transfer to hospital for specialist treatment

Page 204

1. Variance within the data set as a result of a diverse cohort. This may be clinical or methodological if looking at a review article.
2. **a.** Usually, utilise computer-generated lists to assign participants a random number and then assign a treatment option to that number
   b. Do not follow any set pattern
   c. The most commonly used method for randomisation
   d. Can create unequal groups especially in smaller studies
3. False negative

Page 213

1. Site, onset, character, radiation, alleviating factors, timing, exacerbating factors, severity
2. When you want to attain the patient's viewpoint on what is going on

Page 240

1. Coagulopathy, hypothermia, acidosis
2. $KE = \frac{1}{2}mv^2$
3. The greater the energy transferred the greater the risk of injury

Page 249

1. Hypovolaemia, oxygen, tension pneumothorax, tamponade
2. Bone is 'shattered' into multiple pieces
3. **a.** No posterior midline C-spine tenderness
   b. No evidence of intoxication
   c. The normal level of alertness
   d. No focal neurological deficit
   e. No painful distracting injuries

Page 253

1. **a.** True
   b. False, it must first be metabolised
   c. True
2. **a.** Drugs may be less well absorbed if they require bile salts for absorption
   b. Liver failure may create new fluid compartments. Water-soluble drugs may be distributed into these spaces

    c. Chronic liver failure may result in reduced plasma protein levels
       i. Reduced protein binding sites
       ii. Increased free molecules
       iii. Potential for increased efficacy of medications beyond expected
    d. Reduced or delays metabolism of medications

3.   **a.** Actions of common drugs may be unpredictable in the elderly
    b. Reduced number of and efficacy of drug receptors
    c. Increased affinity for opiates and benzodiazepines
    d. Lower physiological reserve to cope with the effects of medications
    e. Drugs will have a narrower therapeutic window
    f. Uncertain absorption of oral medications
    g. Delayed gastric emptying may delay the onset of oral medication
    h. Variable 1st pass metabolism
    i. The decrease in plasma protein, therefore, reduced protein binding of medications
    j. Changes in distribution due to body fat and muscle variations
    k. Reduced hepatic metabolism
    l. Decreased renal excretion therefore drugs may stay within the body for longer
    m. Smaller volumes of fluid may be required to cause fluid overload states

Page 258

1. Positive results are more likely to be published than negative
2. With an asterisk.

Page locators in **bold** indicate tables. Page locators in *italics* indicate figures. This index uses letter-by-letter alphabetization.